Blind Spots

BLIND SPOTS

WHEN MEDICINE GETS IT WRONG, AND WHAT IT MEANS FOR OUR HEALTH

MARTY MAKARY, MD

THORNDIKE PRESS
A part of Gale, a Cengage Company

GALE
A Cengage Company

GALE
A Cengage Company

Thorndike Press, a part of Gale, a Cengage Company.

Thorndike Press® Large Print Nonfiction.

The text of this Large Print edition is unabridged.

Other aspects of the book may vary from the original edition.

Set in 16 pt. Plantin.

LIBRARY OF CONGRESS CIP DATA ON FILE.
CATALOGUING IN PUBLICATION FOR THIS BOOK
IS AVAILABLE FROM THE LIBRARY OF CONGRESS.

ISBN-13: 978-1-4205-2284-6 (hardcover alk. paper)

Published in 2025 by arrangement with Bloomsbury Publishing Inc.

Print Number: 1 Print Year: 2025
Printed in Mexico

Dedicated to my editor Marshall Allen, who unexpectedly passed away a few months before this book's release. Thank you to Marshall for believing in this project, mentoring me in journalism, and being such a great friend. I'm not sure why the good Lord called you home early but many of us will miss you dearly. You dedicated your life to being a voice for the voiceless and challenging corporate interests using the sunlight of investigative journalism. Your articles and recent book made the world a better place and inspired many of us. I hope this book's rollout will honor your dedication to shaping it with me.

And to my father, who dedicated his life to applying the ever-evolving science of hematology to his patients and taught me that it's always okay to ask questions.

PUBLISHER'S NOTE

This a work of nonfiction. However, the names and identifying characteristics of individuals who are identified only by a first name or an initial have been changed to protect their privacy. Any similarity between an individual identified by a fictional first name or initial and any real individual is strictly coincidental.

This book is not intended to provide medical advice to individual readers. To obtain medical advice, the reader should consult a medical professional who will dispense advice based upon each reader's medical history and current medical condition.

CONTENTS

PREFACE 11

1. The Salem Peanut Trial: *How experts created an epidemic* . 21

2. OMG HRT: *The untold story of hormone replacement therapy* . . . 50

3. "No Downsides to Antibiotics": *Except carpet-bombing the microbiome* 88

4. My Uncle Sam Loves Eggs: *The truth about cholesterol* . . . 126

5. True Believers: *Why we resist new ideas* 166

6. Bad Blood: *How the medical establishment actually works* . . . 186

7. A Warm Welcome: *Rethinking how we bring babies into the world* . . 217

8. Challenging Certainty: *The true origin of ovarian cancer* 255

9. Silicone Valley: *Breast implants, autoimmune diseases, and the opioid crisis* 280

10. A Comedy of Errors: *A short history of medical groupthink* . . 304

11. A Culture of Obedience: *The battle for civil discourse* 328

12. Imagine: *What else are we getting wrong?* 367

ACKNOWLEDGMENTS 417

NOTES 419

A NOTE ON THE AUTHOR. . . 497

PREFACE

"Just memorize it for the exam," a medical school classmate would often tell me every time I questioned something. I never liked the hot-dog-eating-contest method of learning. Sure, I liked memorizing emergency procedures and drugs, but the forced memorization and regurgitation of things like the Krebs cycle was mind-numbing. I was much more interested in talking about medicine's giant blind spots. There seemed to be a lot of them — things that made no sense but that we all did anyway.

For example, why did we have a nightly ritual in the hospital of startling patients in their deep sleep, quickly sticking them with a needle to draw their blood, and then running away like we just poked a hibernating bear? When I first witnessed it in training, I asked if I could be a conscientious objector. The great irony was that practically *everybody* in the hospital seemed to know that most of those daily tests were unnecessary, except the patient. In some instances, the only lab result that changed was their blood level — because we were extracting it so frequently.

I was also perplexed by how we responded to hungry patients who begged us for food. We'd feed them small portions of Jell-O and flavorless processed food, a human rights violation by some definitions. When we did give them something with flavor, it was the kind of junk food we'd normally scold people for eating at home. On one occasion, a week after a lady was admitted to the hospital with an infection, my attending physician asked me why she was deteriorating despite her infection improving. I gave my honest assessment: "Sir, the patient came in with one medical illness and then we hit her with two more — sleep deprivation and malnutrition."

People often ask me if artificial intelligence — AI — will help me as a doctor and ultimately transform medicine. I often reply that we don't need "AI," we just need "I."

Groupthink — the human tendency to follow a crowd and not think independently — often creates an illusion of consensus. As a Johns Hopkins physician and researcher, I have visited hundreds of hospitals and medical conferences around the country where I've had the privilege of meeting smart doctors who are challenging modern medicine's deeply held assumptions.

This book may change your life. It did mine. You may forever view everything from menopause to microbiome health differently. You may also develop a reflex to ask for the underlying evidence or rationale to support a health recommendation (e.g., adults should drink three glasses of cow's milk daily) before you blindly abide by it. Having spent many hours with top doctors sorting scientific evidence from opinion on some of today's biggest health questions, I realize that much of what the public is told about health is medical dogma — an idea or practice given incontrovertible authority because someone decreed it to be true based on a gut feeling.

This book is about the latest scientific research on health topics we are not talking about, but should be talking about. Taking the role of a physician-journalist, I was blown away by what I had uncovered. Part of me wondered why this stuff is not taught in medical school. You'll join my conversations with true medical geniuses who have uncovered important truths. Our conversations felt momentous — and I worked hard to distill the "take-home messages" and translate them into plain English. Many of these experts have made groundbreaking discoveries, but their work has not yet been disseminated widely. As you read about them, you may wonder how it's possible that effective ways to prevent problems ranging from peanut allergies and bone fractures to Alzheimer's and cancer are not widely known. At times, I could hardly believe what I was hearing. The research breakthroughs I investigated have largely been underappreciated. I felt compelled to write this book because too few people know about them, even in the medical community.

If you're willing to keep an open mind, as I was challenged to, when you finish this book you will have a whole new perspective on health.

After the initial chapters, we'll pause and examine the human psychology of why we resist new ideas. You'll learn the mechanics of how our minds process new information when it conflicts with what we previously thought to be true. The human brain can do amazing things: feel extreme compassion, comprehend advanced mathematics, and house the seat of the soul. But when it comes to receiving new information that conflicts with old information, it's predictably lazy.

No one studied this principle better than Dr. Leon Festinger. As you'll observe, his milestone psychology experiments showed that humans automatically default to rejecting new information or reframing it in order to ensure that old information in the brain remains true. It's a subconscious effort to avoid the mental distress, or cognitive dissonance, of holding two conflicting ideas at the same time.

Being open to new ideas makes one smarter, less prickly, and more affable — key ingredients of success in life. Being aware of this can result in better relationships, a greater likelihood of promotion, and, when it comes to health, a greater chance of discovering truth. Dr. Festinger teaches us that being open to new ideas requires active mental work to temporarily suspend our prior beliefs as we consider the merits of new ones. Failing to recognize that this is an active process helps explain how good people can become close-minded, and even hostile to new information. I see it every day in business, in politics, and in medicine. It's everywhere.

Despite the tribalism in society today, I'm ultimately optimistic about the future of health care. Today's young innovators — students and residents — are rejecting the broken system they are inheriting.

They see the futility of medicating every problem in society and are quick to call out the medicalization of ordinary life. They have zero interest in getting on the hamster wheel of medicine, seeing patients in hurried 15-minute visits, and spending their nights and weekends obediently billing and coding. I'm inspired that for many, money is not their motivation. They're driven by a thirst for social justice. They are not dismayed when we question conventional thinking. It energizes them.

Together we are asking new questions that challenge current medical dogma. For example, can we treat Type 2 diabetes with cooking classes instead of just prescribing insulin? Can we talk about school lunch programs, not just giving children Ozempic? Can we treat the epidemic of loneliness by fostering communities, instead of simply prescribing endless antidepressants? The current system isn't working. It's time to create a national discussion that challenges the conventional thinking.

That's precisely how we can leapfrog out of today's stagnant state of health care.

You'll notice a pattern as we examine some of modern medicine's biggest health recommendations. When we use sound scientific studies to make recommendations, we shine

— and help a lot of people. But when we wing it and issue recommendations based on opinion, we have a lousy track record. Sometimes you'll see that consensus is not driven by science, but by peer pressure.

In doing the research for this book, I often started my conversations with experts by explaining that I was writing about the topic of medical dogma. Then I'd ask if they knew of medical recommendations that are unproven or have been proven wrong yet are still pushed today. I thought there'd be a slim chance they'd be able to think of something in their specialty. Boy, was I wrong. As soon as I asked the question, the floodgates opened. The doctors would unload, sharing example after example of medical groupthink today gone awry. Our conversations were so animated it was hard to leave some of the interviews. In a few, I took on the role of therapist for doctors who had raised objections within their professional medical society but had been ignored. The dogma list became so long, I actually got scared for a moment and wondered, *Is there anything we do right?*

Of course there is. I see it every time I'm in the operating room or hear of a person beating cancer. Smallpox has been eradicated and childbirth has gone from being a leading cause of death among women to a safe procedure. While researching this book I was also inspired by how sophisticated medicine has become.

The purpose of this book is not to make you cynical about the medical profession (if you're bleeding, please do whatever a doctor tells you). Instead, my goal is to increase public trust by restoring faith in the scientific process itself.

Each chapter presents a different perspective on how smart people can succumb to bandwagon thinking. Each chapter also profiles bold innovators who are going against the grain to show us the truth. Between stories, we'll take a step back to examine the culture of medicine. We'll also explore the newest areas of medical research, including topics like food and longevity.

You may think that the era of medical dogma is long gone. That we are enlightened now! And that today's medical care is universally bolstered by rigorous scientific methodology. But the current wave of major medical recommendations being overturned by good science would suggest that medical dogma is still ubiquitous.

Modern medicine's track record of getting big health recommendations wrong begs the question: What else are we doing today that could be wrong?

Interpreting research objectively is the next big frontier of health care. Simply accepting medical dogma — such as “opioids are nonaddictive” — because experts say so has proven catastrophic. In the case of opioids, the medical-industrial complex steamrolled over early research on addiction, creating an epidemic that killed over a million Americans and cost billions. Parallels could be made to how medical experts demonized natural fat in food, driving people to processed carbohydrates as obesity rates soared, and liberally prescribed antibiotics, altering the gut health of a generation. It begs the question: Could it be that many of our modern-day health crises are caused by the hubris of the medical establishment?

We can enact health care reform, close health disparities, and give every American gold-plated health insurance, but if we continue to recklessly issue health recommendations based on an illusion of consensus instead of proper science, we’ll continue to struggle and waste billions.

Our course correction begins with the real story on health, separating dogma from evidence. That means asking good questions. Questioning assumptions should not be viewed as a threat. It’s the very way we find truth.

CHAPTER 1

The Salem Peanut Trial

How experts created an epidemic

There must be no barriers to freedom of inquiry. There is no place for dogma in science. The scientist is free, and must be free to ask any question, to doubt any assertion, to seek for any evidence, to correct any errors.

— J. Robert Oppenheimer

"Hi, my name is Chase, and I'll be your waiter. Does anyone at the table have a nut allergy?"

My two Johns Hopkins students from Africa, Asonganyi Aminkeng and Faith Magwenzi, looked at each other, perplexed.

"What is it with the peanut allergies here?" Asonganyi asked me. "Ever since I landed at JFK from Cameroon, I noticed a food apartheid — food packages either read 'Contains Tree Nuts' or 'Contains No Tree Nuts.' "

Asonganyi told me that even on his connecting flight to Baltimore, the flight attendant had made an announcement: "We have someone on the plane with a peanut allergy, so please try not to eat peanuts." And on his first day at Johns Hopkins, a classmate invited him to dinner. The invite went something like this: 1) Would you like to come over for dinner; and 2) do you have a peanut or other allergy?

"What's going on here?" Asonganyi asked with a big smile. "We have no peanut allergies in Africa."

Faith, who had flown in from Zimbabwe, nodded in agreement.

I looked at them and smiled. "In Egypt, where my family is from, we don't have peanut allergies either," I said. "Welcome to America. Peanut allergies are real and can be life-threatening here."

Their observation reminded me of when my friend's school banned peanuts from the campus. School administrators actually inquired with security authorities if metal detectors could detect a peanut. And then one day there was an "emergency." A peanut was found on the floor of a school bus. It was like discovering an IED in Iraq. The kids were ordered to quietly exit the bus single-file until someone arrived to "decontaminate" the bus. Luckily, the peanut did not detonate and harm the public.

How did we get here?

In 1999, researchers at Mount Sinai Hospital estimated the incidence of peanut allergies in children to be 0.6%. Most were mild.[1] Then starting in the year 2000, the prevalence began to surge. Doctors began to notice that more and more children affected had severe allergies.[2]

Let me share with you the real story behind the rapid growth of this epidemic.

The 1990s was the decade of peanut allergy panic. The media covered children who died of a peanut allergy and doctors began writing more about the issue, speculating on the growing rate of the problem.[3] The American Academy of Pediatrics (AAP) wanted to respond by telling parents what they should do to protect their kids. There was just one problem: They didn't know what precautions, if any, parents should take. Rather than admit that, in the year 2000 the AAP issued a recommendation for children 0 to 3 years old and pregnant and lactating mothers to avoid all peanuts if any child was considered to be at high risk for developing an allergy.[4]

The AAP committee mimicked what the UK health department had recommended two years earlier: total peanut abstinence.[5] The recommendation was technically for high-risk children but the AAP authors acknowledged that "the ability to determine which infants are high risk is imperfect." Having a family member with any allergy or asthma could qualify as "high-risk" using the strictest interpretation. And many well-meaning pediatricians and parents read the recommendation and thought, *Why take chances?* Instantly, pediatricians adopted a simple mnemonic to teach all parents in their offices: "Remember 1-2-3. Age 1: start milk. Age 2: start eggs. Age 3: start peanuts." A generation of pediatricians was indoctrinated with this mantra.

I did a close read of that 1998 UK health department recommendation to see if it cited any scientific studies to back up the decree. I found one sentence stating that moms who eat peanuts are more likely to have children with peanut allergies. In other words, it blamed the moms. The report cited a 1996 *British Medical Journal* (*BMJ*) study.[6] So I pulled that up and took a close look.

I couldn't believe it.

The actual data did *not* find an association between pregnant moms eating peanuts and a child's peanut allergy. But that didn't matter: The train had left the station.

How could "experts" make a recommendation citing a study that did not even support the recommendation?

Bewildered by how the study seemed so badly misconstrued, I called its lead author, Dr. Jonathan Hourihane, a professor of pediatrics in Dublin, Ireland. He shared the same frustration and told me he had opposed the peanut avoidance guideline when it came out. "It's ridiculous," he told me. "It's not what I wanted people to believe."

I specifically asked him how he felt about his study being used as the source to justify the sweeping recommendation. "I felt crossed," he responded, using a little UK slang for feeling betrayed. He had not been consulted on the national guideline.

The 2000 AAP guideline was published in the specialty's top journal, *Pediatrics,* activating many pediatricians to evangelize mothers when they brought their babies in for a checkup. Doctors and public health leaders had their new marching orders. Within months, a mass public education crusade was in full swing and mothers, doing what they thought was best for their children, responded by following the instructions to protect their children.

But despite these efforts, things got worse. By 2004, it was clear that the rate of peanut allergies was going the wrong way. Peanut allergies soared. More concerning, extreme peanut allergies, which can be life-threatening, became commonplace in America.

Suddenly, emergency department visits for peanut anaphylaxis — a life-threatening allergic swelling of the airways — skyrocketed, and schools began enacting peanut bans. By 2007, 18% of Virginia schools had banned peanuts altogether. And in 2016, the Parkway School District in St. Louis County, Missouri, reported 957 students with documented life-threatening food allergies, most of which were to peanuts. The rate had increased 50% from just six years prior, and more than 1,000% from a prior generation.

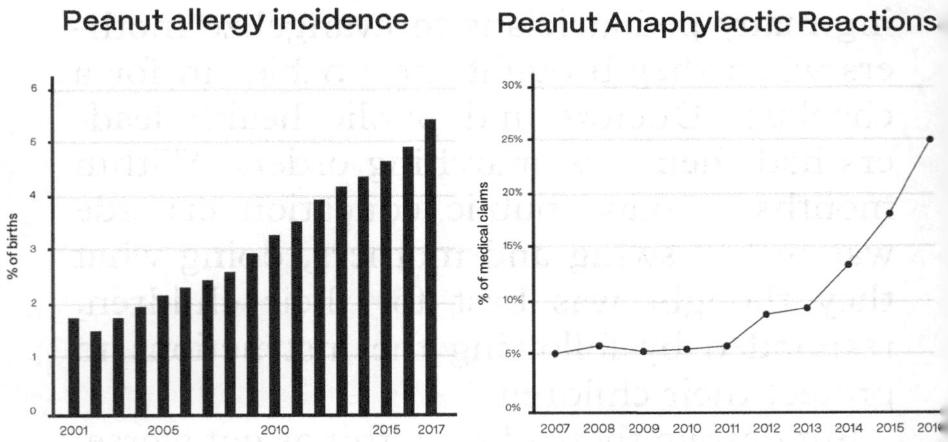

The Peanut Allergy Epidemic: (Left) Estimated number of peanut allergie[s] per birth in the U.S. following the American Academy of Pediatrics recommendation for young children to avoid peanuts issued in the year 2000. (Right) Anaphylactic reactions to peanuts.

(M. Motosue et al., *Annals of Allergy, Asthma & Immunology,* 2018; FAIR Health)

As things got worse, many public health leaders doubled down. If only every parent would comply with the pediatrics association guideline, they thought, we as a country could finally beat down peanut allergies and win the war. The dogma became a self-licking ice cream cone.

But the groupthink could not have been more wrong.

Swimming Against the Current

Dr. Stephen Combs is a salt-of-the-earth pediatrician in rural East Tennessee. At one point, the other pediatricians in Dr. Combs's group noticed something unique about his patients. None of them had peanut allergies. This despite the fact that his colleagues were seeing more and more kids with peanut allergies in their practices. What was going on?

I was curious to learn more about his impressive track record, so I traveled to the beautiful rolling hills of Johnson City, Tennessee, to visit him. (I often learn a lot when I get outside of the bubble of my urban university hospital.)

I discovered that all the pediatricians in Dr. Combs's group were as impressive as he was: making house calls, staying late to see patients, and educating parents on how to raise healthy children. They all practiced pediatrics the same way.

Except for one thing.

Dr. Combs had never followed the AAP guideline for young children to avoid peanuts. The reason for his defiance was simple. Dr. Combs did his residency at Duke Medical Center in North Carolina, where he trained under world-famous pediatric immunologist Dr. Rebecca Buckley. When the AAP guideline came out in 2000 with a big splash, Dr. Buckley recognized that it violated a basic principle of immunology known as immune tolerance: the body's natural way of accepting foreign molecules present early in life. It's like the dirt theory, whereby newborns exposed to dirt, dander, and germs may then have lower allergy and asthma risks.[7] Dr. Buckley confidently told her students and residents, including Dr. Combs, to ignore the AAP recommendation, and in fact, to do the opposite. She explained that peanut abstinence doesn't *prevent* peanut allergies, it *causes* them.

Her explanation turned out to be prophetic.

Since his training with Dr. Buckley, Dr. Combs has consistently instructed parents to introduce a touch of peanut butter (mixed with water to avoid a choking risk) as soon as a child is able to eat it. To this day, the thousands of children in East Tennessee lucky enough to have Dr. Combs as their pediatrician do not have peanut allergies.

Extrapolating the principle to other potential allergens, Dr. Combs also encouraged the early introduction of eggs, milk, strawberries, and even early exposure to dogs and cats. As a result, the children in his practice rarely developed an allergy to these things, and when they did, it was mild.

An Embarrassingly Simple Study

Dr. Buckley and her trainees were not alone in bucking the AAP's guidance. In fact, many experts in immunology had long known of mouse studies showing that avoiding certain foods triggers allergies to those foods. But the laboratory immunology community was largely disconnected from the clinical allergist and the pediatric community.

Dr. Gideon Lack, a pediatric allergist and immunologist in London, challenged the UK guideline. It "was not evidence-based," he wrote in *The Lancet* in 1998. "Public-health measures may have unintended effects . . . they could increase the prevalence of peanut allergy."[8]

Two years later, the same year the AAP issued their peanut avoidance recommendation, he was giving a lecture in Israel on allergies and asked the roughly 200 pediatricians in the audience, "How many of you are seeing kids with a peanut allergy?"

Only two or three raised their hands. Back in London, nearly every pediatrician had raised their hand to the same question.

Startled by the discrepancy, he had a Eureka moment. Many Israeli infants are fed a peanut-based food called Bamba. To him, it was no coincidence.

Dr. Lack quickly assembled researchers in Tel Aviv and Jerusalem to launch a formal study. They found that Jewish children in Israel had one tenth the rate of peanut allergies compared to Jewish children in the UK, suggesting it was not a genetic predisposition, as the medical establishment had assumed.[9] Lack and his Israeli colleagues titled their publication "Early Consumption of Peanuts in Infancy Is Associated with a Low Prevalence of Peanut Allergy."

However, their publication in 2008 was not enough to uproot the groupthink. Avoiding peanuts had been the correct answer on medical school tests and board exams, which were written and administered by the American Board of Pediatrics. Many in the medical community dismissed Dr. Lack's findings and continued to insist that young children avoid peanuts. For nearly a decade after AAP's peanut avoidance recommendation, neither the National Institutes of Health's (NIH's) National Institute of Allergy and Infectious Diseases (NIAID) nor other institutions would fund a robust study to evaluate the recommendation, to see if it was helping or hurting children.

But things were getting worse. The more health officials implored parents to follow the recommendation, the worse peanut allergies got. The number of children going to the emergency department because of peanut allergies tripled in just one decade (2005–14).[10] It spread like a virus. By 2019, one report estimated that 1 in every 18 American children had a peanut allergy.[11] Schools continued to ban peanuts and regulators met to purge peanuts from childhood snacks as EpiPen sales soared. Pharma exploited the situation by price-gouging the desperate parents and schools. Mylan Pharmaceuticals jacked up the price of an EpiPen from $100 to $600 in the U.S. (It's $30 in some countries.)[12]

The AAP recommendation had created a vicious cycle. The more prevalent peanut allergies became, the more people avoided peanuts for young children. This, in turn, caused more peanut allergies. Tunnel-vision thinking had created a nightmare scenario for which the only possible solution seemed to be the total eradication of peanuts from the planet.

As things got worse, a dissenting Dr. Lack decided to conduct the study to end all studies — a clinical trial randomizing infants to peanut exposure (at 4–11 months of age) versus no peanut exposure. He found that early peanut exposure resulted in an 86% reduction in peanut allergies by the time the child reached age 5 compared to children who followed the AAP recommendation.[13] He blasted his findings to the world in a *New England Journal of Medicine* publication in 2015, finally proving what immunologists like Dr. Buckley had known for decades: Peanut abstinence causes peanut allergies. It was now undeniable; the AAP had it backward.

I reached out to Dr. Lack and had breakfast with him when he was traveling to Washington, D.C., for a medical conference in 2024. He told me that his initial hypothesis had been based on an early observation as a pediatrician that kids who got their ears pierced sometimes developed a nickel allergy around the piercing. But kids who had orthodontics didn't. He realized that kids with orthodontics had prior exposure to nickel in the braces, making them immune. This observation was consistent with the concept of "oral tolerance" that he'd studied in mice experiments conducted at the University of Colorado in the 1990s.

He also had an interesting observation from his childhood that reminded him that conventional wisdom can change. His grandfather had a heart attack, which doctors treated with strict bed rest — a recommendation that was eventually replaced with cardiac rehab exercise. As a 6-year-old, Dr. Lack recalled that his grandfather was not allowed to leave his bed. The family members had to take him his meals. His doctors managed his damaged heart by weakening it further.

"In science, we tend to get in a rut and then dig in," he told me. "We have to be open-minded."

Dr. Lack is now recognized as a hero in the field of allergy. But when he did his big study, he was heavily criticized. The 100% breast-feeding purists called him "anti-breast-feeding" for saying a slurry of food bits should be introduced to infants. But Dr. Lack wasn't anti-breast-feeding at all. Quite the opposite! Breast-feeding was entirely compatible with introducing a touch of peanut butter and other foods at 3 to 6 months of age. He had to withstand other criticism.

"I was accused of unethical behavior. There was huge pressure to stop the study," he told me. "Testing the hypothesis was seen as unethical because it seemed preposterous."

Some also worried that peanuts could cause obesity because they are high in saturated fat (a topic we'll explore soon in chapter 4, "My Uncle Sam Loves Eggs").

It would take the AAP two years after Dr. Lack's randomized trial was published to reverse its 2000 guidance for pediatricians and parents.[14] It would also take two years for the NIH's NIAID division to issue a report supporting the reversal.[15]

Did they really need two years? Where was the sense of deep remorse? The affected families deserved to have the medical establishment move with a sense of urgency to correct their recommendation immediately following Dr. Lack's definitive study. Dr. Hugh Sampson, another trainee of Rebecca Buckley, led the NIAID report that undid the recommendation. He told me that working with the government agency was frustrating. Dr. Sampson is one of the country's leading allergists. When I asked him what he thought about the entire saga, he told me, "The food allergy community has been appropriately chastised [for getting the peanut recommendation wrong]."

An entire generation — millions of children — had been harmed by groupthink, and many still are feeling the effects. Now, at least the faucet of bad advice was turned off.

My Friend

The 2015 study had been a bombshell. I called one of my best friends from medical school, Dr. Drew White, now an allergist at the Scripps Clinic in San Diego, to ask him how it has been received. "It's an impressive study," he said. "After it came out, we immediately thought, 'How are we going to fix this giant mess?'" The AAP's absolutism in 2000 had made the recommendation hard to walk back. Drew and I agreed: The AAP should have originally said something like, "We're not sure." At least that would have been honest.

Tragically, to this day, many parents still believe they should avoid peanuts for their infants and toddlers. The peanut abstinence recommendation had been so vigorous for so long, it's what people still remember.

There are effective treatments that involve slowly reintroducing small doses of peanuts with powerful medications to suppress a child's immune response. Sadly, that's too much of a hardship or too expensive for some people who find it easier to manage their allergy by avoiding peanuts.

During the 15 years between the AAP guideline and Dr. Lack's definitive study, parents who allowed their young children to eat peanut products were viewed almost like criminals by some in the medical establishment and society at large. Scolding and public shaming ensued. Parents out of compliance with the AAP guideline were viewed as idiots who arrogantly defied science.[16]

My friend Drew and I discussed how we wished the definitive study had been conducted back in the 1990s — before AAP's misguided recommendation. It's not a cash-poor organization. The AAP brought in $137 million in 2022[17] from member dues ($692/year per board-certified pediatrician), pharma, baby formula companies, and other sources. Lives could have been saved if the peanut avoidance dogma had not been put forward. Funding a research study to answer the big peanut-allergy question *before* issuing sweeping recommendations would have spared countless families tremendous pain and avoided billions in medical expenses. Dr. Lack's 2015 study was game-changing, but it was also a very basic randomized trial involving 640 children. It was embarrassingly simple.

Deaths from peanut allergies are real. And living with one can be terrifying. Compounding the tragedy is knowing that the current epidemic of peanut allergies was largely avoidable. To understand more about what it's like to live with a severe peanut allergy, I met with a few families who live with one.

A young girl named Charley made the biggest impression on me. When Charley was born at the height of the peanut abstinence dogma, in 2009, her mom, Jen, tried to do everything right in raising her little girl. For example, she obeyed the guidance in *Consumer Reports* to replace a bike helmet every time it fell to the ground in case it had a small crack. So when it came to peanut products, she did a lot of research, especially since Charley had some skin eczema when she was a 1-year-old. "Let's stop all peanuts," her pediatrician told her, in compliance with the AAP guideline. To be sure, Jen, who happened to be a school nurse herself, consulted with a second pediatrician. Her husband, Shane, called a family friend in Kentucky who was a newly minted pediatrician.

"Everyone said the same thing," Jen and Shane told me. So the parents meticulously complied with total peanut abstinence. However, within months, little Charley started getting sick a lot. It began with a diagnosis of asthma and progressed to a severe peanut allergy. Within years, even being near peanuts without touching them could trigger a reaction in which her throat swelled and she couldn't breathe. Jen and Shane told me they had a few close calls, and that the fear of being exposed created a lot of anxiety in their daughter's life.

The hardest part, they told me, was when people downplayed Charley's nut allergy. They shared how hard it is to take their daughter out for ice cream. They have to ask the server (sometimes a high schooler) to please use a fresh scooper and pull ice cream from an unopened bin to prevent any cross-contamination from the pistachio bin. They have to be vigilant, or they risk an emergency. Sometimes the ice-cream server argues with them, insisting that rinsing the scooper is sufficient or all they can do. This level of oversight can convert a nice evening out into a nightmare for the family. The couple became so tired of arguing with food establishments, they considered starting a business to educate restaurants and maybe even create a seal for allergy-friendly restaurants. Some teenagers with severe allergies have never been to a restaurant in their life.

Today, Charley is far down the path of a desensitization program. Doctors have her eating a few peanut M&M's most nights along with medication to reduce her allergy. But even today, each time she eats the peanuts, her body suffers a mini reaction that gives her a stomachache. She hates doing it. She's asked to stop, but her doctors have told her she needs to keep at it to downgrade her allergy from life-threatening to non-life-threatening. They are also looking into newer treatments that have become available.

Jen and Shane never imagined they could have been getting bad advice from their trusted pediatricians. "You have all these people you respect and went to medical school saying the same thing," Jen told me. "You just don't question that they could be wrong."

Shane was more blunt: "I feel 100% dumbfounded that my poor kid is living with this because of one bad document," he said, referring to the 2000 AAP recommendation. "I'm looking at my kid and feel sad for her because she has to live in fear because we got misinformation. You would assume that doctors would do their own research and not just blindly follow."

The couple also expressed feeling that the medical profession was not honest. The flawed peanut abstinence idea had been recommended with the same vigor as other proven recommendations. The pair had no way of knowing that one was made-up, and the others were based on solid evidence.

I listened to Shane's frustration with sorrow because I knew that back in 2000, scientists in the immunology community knew the truth about early exposure, and they'd had strong data to support it. But they were not included in the small committee that had issued the AAP recommendation. Dr. Sampson, the influential allergist, explained to me the sad reality of how medicine can be siloed. "People from the immunology community didn't really interact with the clinical allergy or nutrition community," he said. Furthermore, food allergy "was not a respected specialty," he added. "The sense in the pediatric hierarchy was that allergy was not that important and not a real science."

After spending time with Charley's family, the rise in peanut allergies in the U.S. exacerbated by the flawed AAP recommendation was no longer just a chart in my mind, it was a vivid tragedy.

To better understand the scope of the problem, I reached out to Dr. Robin Wallin, director of school health services at Alexandria, Virginia, public schools, just outside of Washington, D.C. Given the high prevalence of peanut allergies at the school (practically every classroom has a child with one), the school today discourages the use of food for celebrations like birthdays and holidays.

While celebrations in classrooms were disappearing, Dr. Wallin explained to me that the budget for EpiPens had exploded. They are everywhere, cost hundreds of dollars each, and have to be restocked each year because they expire. Interestingly, she mentioned to me that while peanut allergies are prevalent, she hardly ever sees them among the many immigrant children in the school district. Many of their home countries were spared the AAP dogma that spread throughout the U.S.

Where Did the Absolutists Go?

We all make mistakes, but when we do, it's important to take responsibility for them. In medicine, it's vital. Doing so enables us to set up processes to prevent future mistakes. It's also important to apologize to the people harmed by the error. In fact, it's a crucial part of the healing process and builds trust.

I reached out to the AAP committee that had recommended peanut avoidance back in 2000. By their credentials, many appeared to be in the field of nutrition. None appeared to be experts in immunology. The committee was comprised of a small core group of seven physicians and nine representatives from the Centers for Disease Control (CDC), the Food and Drug Administration (FDA), the NIH, the U.S. Department of Agriculture, the American Dietetic Association, and others. Since the publication of their recommendations, none have expressed regret or apologized. Most went on to receive national awards and academic promotions. I contacted all of them for a comment.

Two of the seven committee members got back to me. One acknowledged to me that the recommendation in the year 2000 came from a previous AAP handbook on nutrition. "There was an internal policy that all AAP recommendations had to be consistent. It was old dogma, perpetuated." In other words, protecting the institution was more important than letting the public see alternative viewpoints.

Another committee member responded by telling me that he is not an allergist. "Have never treated any children for peanut allergy but strongly believe early exposure is the way to go," he wrote. When I spoke with him by

Zoom, he told me that he had had little to do with the guideline but acknowledged "it became dogma." He added, "Any recommendation based on expert *opinion* should be taken with a grain of salt."

Sadly, remnants of the peanut avoidance recommendation still linger. The U.S. food program known as the Special Supplemental Nutrition Program for Women, Infants, and Children (WIC) excludes peanut butter from the list of foods covered for infants. This, despite children who are eligible for the WIC program being at a much higher risk of developing peanut allergies, and thus standing to benefit the most from the early introduction. I spoke with Dr. Lack about this issue. "The WIC program provides a unique public health opportunity to prevent peanut allergy. If peanut butter was to be one of the foods included, it could prevent more than 50% of new cases of peanut allergy every year," he said. This is a modern-day scandal that's still ongoing. I'm raising the issue to members of Congress now, hoping the next announcement about foods covered by WIC will include peanut butter for infants.

I asked Harvard pediatric immunologist Dr. Talal Chatila about the peanut epidemic of the last two and a half decades. He acknowledged that there are multiple factors to consider but that when you push peanut avoidance as boldly as it was pushed, "you end up creating a monster."

On May 28, 2024, Dr. Lack published the long-term outcomes of the children who had participated in his original study. "Peanut consumption, starting in infancy and continuing to age 5 years, provided lasting tolerance to peanut into adolescence," he and his colleagues concluded in the *New England Journal*.[18]

To this day, the UK and the U.S. continue to have the worst peanut allergy problems in the world.

Ending Starvation

The United States also exported its peanut misinformation. Peanuts are rich in protein, fiber, healthy fats, vitamins, and minerals, making them an ideal food to address world hunger. They do not require refrigeration for storage and transportation, and they can be mixed with water for hydration and to avoid the risk of airway obstruction. They're also cheap. That's why they've been a miracle food for international relief agencies that have focused on delivering Bamba and other peanut-based foods to the children of the world. Bamba is pretty amazing. It contains no preservatives or food coloring and is enriched with several vitamins. People can live off Bamba and water for a long time. It has been distributed to millions of children around the world and has saved countless lives.

But when American pediatricians recommended against feeding young children any peanut-containing foods in 2000, it presented a dilemma for international relief workers: Did early exposure to peanut products really cause peanut allergies? And if so, was it worth the risk to prevent starvation deaths?

Some international aid workers were smart enough to see that Africans were eating soups with boiled peanuts starting in infancy and no one seemed to develop a peanut allergy. They pressed ahead with distributing Bamba despite opposition from some U.S. pediatricians.

The U.S. medical establishment was exporting our ignorant dogma about peanut avoidance. For 15 years, smart doctors and immunologists challenging the AAP on this were no match for the powerful trade association and NIAID. Thankfully, Dr. Lack's 2015 study was solid evidence they could not deny. In the end, the early observations of African relief workers were more correct than academic elites.

During those same 15 years when the UK and U.S. recommended peanut avoidance, Asonganyi and Faith's home countries in Africa witnessed no peanut allergies, except among American and UK expats and tourists. I learned from Asonganyi and Faith that they, like many African infants and young children, were transitioned from breast milk by drinking sips of boiled peanut soup. (Incidentally, boiled peanuts are less allergenic than roasted peanuts, which are popular in the U.S.) Their immune systems loved it.

Thanks to good research, peanut-based foods now flourish around the world, addressing world hunger and preventing peanut allergies. In comparing health care systems, Africa prevented disease the right way as Westerners scrambled in fear, stocked with caches of expensive EpiPens.

A Path Forward

The AAP and U.S. public health officials should try a new strategy. They should adopt a national campaign to educate parents on the importance of introducing safe peanut products to infants. They should also encourage people with severe allergies to seek state-of-the art medical treatment. In the past, there was little one could do about a severe peanut allergy except avoidance. Today, doctors can assimilate these children with medical best practices: slowly, frequently, and in a stepwise fashion, reintroducing peanuts. Beginning in 2005, European doctors have treated children with this controlled reintroduction in conjunction with an immune system medication called Xolair (a monoclonal antibody to the IgE "allergy" antibody). *Nineteen years* later, in 2024, the FDA approved the drug for use in the U.S.[19] Stepwise reintroduction is not an instant cure, but over time this therapy can reduce or negate one's dependence on EpiPens for survival.

The story of peanut allergies, to some extent, is mirrored by other food allergies, including eggs and milk. Instead of giving people the wrong advice based on flimsy data, the AAP should have been honest and told parents the correct answer to their question on how to prevent peanut allergies in the year 2000: We don't know. It's one thing to give an opinion, but it's another thing to suggest that an opinion is a scientific truth. As you'll see in the coming chapters, the simple words "We don't know" can often be the right answer.

Trust

When modern medicine issues recommendations based on good scientific studies, we shine. Conversely, when modern medicine rules by opinion and edict, we have an embarrassing track record. In this book, we will explore how some of the biggest recommendations of modern medicine have been reversed, some without the public knowing. The backstories are often jaw-dropping, and the truth is essential to your health.

The most important characteristic of a good doctor is humility. The humility to know their limits, when to tap another doctor for help, and when to say, "I don't know." In my experience, people are forgiving if you are open and honest with them. But they have little tolerance for making statements with strict absolutism when in reality these statements are based upon a gut feeling — or an opinion based on no valid scientific data. The most unforgivable offense for many is when doctors make a strong recommendation based on no scientific data but suggest that it *is* backed up by science. That causes a breakdown in trust.

Dr. Gideon Lack is an international hero. He dared to challenge conventional thinking and ultimately reversed a medical dogma that harmed millions of children. Moreover, he generated the scientific data to do it.

The next time a waiter asks you if anyone at the table has a peanut allergy, you can thank the medical oligarchs who stormed ahead with a recommendation without doing the proper scientific study first or including people from the immunology community. Also, remember that this is a question that waiters in Africa do not need to ask.

CHAPTER 2

OMG HRT

The untold story of hormone replacement therapy

Truth, they say, is all too frequently eclipsed but never extinguished.

— Titus Livius

For most of the 20th century, hormone replacement therapy (HRT) was celebrated as a medical miracle. Millions of women using HRT found relief from the symptoms of menopause. HRT, which is estrogen with or without progesterone, alleviated hot flashes, reduced brain fog and depression, and even helped women sleep better. Not only did women *feel* better on HRT, but studies found they were also less likely to develop Alzheimer's and bone fractures, and they had a 50% lower risk of dying of a heart attack when they started HRT within ten years of menopause.[1] Overall, HRT has been shown to increase a woman's longevity by three years. Millions of women around the world have felt better and lived longer, healthier lives thanks to HRT.

But then in 2002, something happened.

Doctors from the NIH held a press conference to announce a surprising discovery. HRT, they said, causes breast cancer. Their conclusion was based on a 16,608-woman study they had just completed with Harvard and Stanford researchers. "These findings are the first confirmation from a rigorous clinical trial that taking estrogen plus progestin increases the risk of breast cancer," lead author Dr. Jacques Rossouw said, adding that HRT resulted in "a 26% higher incidence of breast cancer." He didn't release any of the study's data but claimed the study had been stopped early because of this concerning finding. The shocking announcement scared women around the world, and doctors, too. HRT was instantly deemed a carcinogen and abandoned.[2] Women flushed their pills down the toilet and doctors stopped prescribing them.

The media clapped like seals congratulating the researchers. Reporters amplified the study's conclusion, even though they had not yet seen the actual data. *Time* magazine put a woman on its cover with an ominous headline: "The Truth about Hormones: Hormone-replacement therapy is riskier than advertised. What's a woman to do?" The researchers were celebrated as savvy medical detectives whose discovery would rescue millions of women from a dreaded cancer.

There was just one problem: The study had NOT shown that HRT causes breast cancer.

The actual publication, which appeared in the *Journal of the American Medical Association* (*JAMA*) one week after the press conference, did not support the headlined conclusion. It reported no statistically significant difference in the rates of breast cancer among the women on HRT compared to those who took a placebo. The authors had misrepresented their data. But amazingly, hardly anyone noticed. The message that HRT causes breast cancer stuck. And that message is still believed by most doctors to this day.

Not everyone drank the Kool-Aid. I was a resident at the time. One of my mentors, known for her impartiality, pointed out to me the massive discrepancy between the study announcement and the published data.

"Is this a Jedi mind trick?" she asked me in disbelief. "This may be the greatest farce in modern medicine."

I asked her to walk me through the data in the publication. She pointed out that the rate of early breast cancer (what we call carcinoma in situ) was stated in the article to be no different with HRT. The rate of invasive breast cancer was slightly higher in the HRT group than the placebo group, less than 1 additional nonfatal breast cancer diagnosis per 1,000 women treated in a year, but given the large size of each group, only a valid statistical test would determine if the difference was real — or just random noise in the data. That's how science is done. It's Research 101. No journal or legitimate scientist would ever accept claims of a higher rate in one group over another group if the statistical test applied found no difference.

I checked the statistical test in the publication. It was a standard test. We call it an "odds ratio confidence interval." When a confidence interval is wide and includes the number 1.0 in the range, it is considered nonsignificant, meaning there is no difference between the groups being tested. *Always*. In this study, the confidence interval was so wide, you could drive a Mack truck through it. More importantly, it also included the number 1.0 in the range.

"Marty, it's amazing," my mentor exclaimed. "The study showing that HRT causes breast cancer does not show that HRT causes breast cancer!"

As time went on, my mentor and I were baffled that no one was speaking up. We wondered when a prominent doctor would finally and publicly point out the false claims made by the NIH researcher. *Surely someone will expose this,* we thought. *There can't be that many people who don't understand statistics.*

0.83-1.92
0.29-2.32
0.32-1.24

Published confidence interval c the adjusted risk of invasive bre cancer for women taking HRT compared to placebo

(JOURNAL OF THE AMERICAN MEDICAL ASSOCIATION, JULY 17, 2002)

We were wrong. The few doctors who spoke up were crowded out. U.S. prescriptions for HRT plummeted by 80%, and they remain low to this day. Tragically, a generation of millions of women were deprived of a life-changing treatment.

A cruel irony came to light in follow-up studies. They found that participants who took estrogen alone had lowered their risk of breast cancer by 23% and lowered their risk of breast cancer death by 40%. That benefit diminished over time after women discontinued HRT.

Yet to my utter amazement, to this day, many doctors still believe that HRT should not be prescribed because it causes breast cancer. If you ask them why, they will almost certainly cite this famous study — the most expensive clinical study in history — known around the world as the Women's Health Initiative (WHI). The NIH had spent approximately $1 billion in taxpayer dollars on the study.

The Incredible Backstory

When I set out to investigate how the WHI debacle happened, doctors close to the study told me I should talk to Dr. Robert Langer, a University of California San Diego epidemiologist and preventive medicine expert who was also a WHI investigator. He has been outspoken about how the WHI lead authors misled the public. I reached out to him to learn more.

When we met, Dr. Langer explained that most of the coauthors of the WHI study had been bamboozled at a meeting held on June 27, 2002, just weeks before the study was published in *JAMA*. He walked into the regularly scheduled biannual meeting of the study's 40 principal investigators (one leader from each participating site) at the beautiful new Sofitel Chicago hotel. They were greeted with pleasantries. They had no idea what was about to hit them.

"Welcome to Chicago," the meeting began. Dr. Langer and a researcher from Hawaii were a bit bleary-eyed coming from western time zones.

"You can throw out the agenda we sent you. Things have changed," they were told. The lead biostatistician went on to explain that the study's independent board recommended stopping the HRT trial. Dr. Langer and the other 39 principal investigators (PIs) were told that a small group of the study's leaders had already written the research article, and it had already been accepted for publication at *JAMA,* the most widely read medical journal in the United States.

"Proof" copies of the article were then handed out to the PIs in the room.

The PIs couldn't believe it. Coauthors are always given ample time to review a paper before it's submitted for publication. The investigators objected, stunned by the highly unusual, top-down approach. They were given 20 minutes to read the study. But as they read it, the researchers pointed out misleading language in the article and spotted problems with its conclusions.

Dr. Rossouw, the head of the entire study, tried to calm the researchers by inviting them to make suggested edits and return their marked-up drafts to him before lunch.

He said he would have a courier run over any changes to the journal's offices, only a few blocks from their meeting in Chicago.

"By noon?" The researchers objected. It was already 10:30 A.M. Most of the PIs didn't bother making edits. But Dr. Langer told me how he and a few others used the next hour to make major revisions to the article. They submitted their edits before the noon deadline. But after lunch, they were informed that the courier had returned with the message: It was too late. The article had already been typeset and printed. The journals were stacked at the warehouse, ready to be shipped.

This meeting was a charade.

The focus of the meeting then turned to the proposed press release, titled: "NHLBI [a division of NIH] Stops Trial of Estrogen Plus Progestin Due to Increased Breast Cancer Risk, Lack of Overall Benefit."[3] The PIs' ire boiled over. Remember, these are respectable researchers with MDs and PhDs. Dr. Langer, the most vocal among them, got into a shouting match with Dr. Rossouw.

"If this is what you put out to the press, there's no turning back," Dr. Langer told him.[4] He explained that breast cancer is the biggest hot-button issue in America, adding that "if you stir baseless fear around something so sensitive, you can't put that genie back in the bottle."

Dr. Langer told me, "Marty, it was clear to me that if that press release was put out there, it was game over. And that's exactly what happened."

Over the next several years, Dr. Langer would take issue with other WHI studies and even resign as a coauthor of some of the papers. "It was obvious that the agenda in subsequent reports was to preserve the storyline and save face, given how large and expensive the study was," he explained. His internal resistance did not go unnoticed.

In 2009, Dr. Langer received an email informing him that he was being removed as chair of a WHI committee and banned from involvement in any future WHI publications on HRT. When he asked why, he received the following email response from a WHI leader:

> The PIs have reached a consensus on interpretation of our data and prefer that our publications not be contradictory.

In other words: *We will not tolerate dissent.*

Reflecting on the ordeal, Dr. Langer wrote in 2017 that "highly unusual circumstances" surrounding the early termination and reporting of the trial resulted in the "misinformation and hysteria" that persists today. In a different medical journal, he said that "good science became distorted and ultimately caused substantial and ongoing harm to women for whom appropriate and beneficial treatment was either stopped or never started."[5] When I spoke with him, he shared with me that being fired from the WHI "was at the time very troubling and stressful. Now I see it as one of my proudest moments."

In 2023, Dr. Langer and others published a detailed article condemning "the WHI's reporting of nonsignificant results as if they were meaningful, a misinterpretation of its own data, and the misleading assertion that the WHI's findings have reduced the incidence of breast cancer in the United States."[6] He and his coauthors concluded that, "A generation of women has been deprived of HT [hormone therapy] largely as a result of this widely publicized misinterpretation of the data."

Why did the study's small group of leaders hide data from their coauthors? It may be because the lead author, Dr. Rossouw, had made up his mind before the study began. He had written six years prior to the WHI publication, "It is time to put the brakes on the hormone bandwagon."[7] Well, he did.

I reached out to Dr. Rossouw at his Maryland home to get his take on what went down at that Chicago meeting. He acknowledged that the publication had been hurried and contentious. "That created some unhappiness," he said. "It created a very uncomfortable meeting . . . but we got over it."

My biggest question was about statistical significance. A finding is either statistically significant, which means we can make medical decisions based on it, or it's not. I asked Dr. Rossouw point blank: Was the breast cancer link in his study statistically significant?

"It touched on significance but wasn't quite significant," he replied. "It was nominally significant. It was not significant after being adjusted for multiple looks at the data."

Huh? What a strange way to acknowledge that it was not. I have never heard someone spin a nonsignificant result like that before in my career. It made no sense. I then asked him if his trial or any trial has ever shown that HRT was associated with an increase in mortality due to breast cancer. He said no.

Amazing.

Months after the publication of the WHI's HRT study, a noted oncologist, Dr. Avrum

Bluming, invited one of the three lead investigators, Dr. Rowan Chlebowski, to give a lecture at California's Medical Center of Tarzana. Dr. Bluming told me the audience was not impressed by the non-statistically significant "evidence" presented.

During the Q&A portion after Dr. Chlebowski's lecture, a physician in the audience challenged the WHI investigator, politely asking, "About your claim of the increased risk of breast cancer for women on HRT, I was under the impression that if the confidence interval included the number one, that it was not particularly meaningful."

Dr. Chlebowski responded saying, "Yeah, yeah, you know, that's right. And you know what happens? What happens is, if it's an important question and if it's a big study . . . and you can't do it again because it costs too much money, then they'll say that's the best data there is and then . . . the statistical police have to leave the room."[8]

The audience was silent, flabbergasted by the glib dismissal of universally accepted research standards. There were no more questions.

Dr. Garnet Anderson, the study's statistician, had gone on record saying that when it's an issue as important to women as breast cancer, we intentionally set the bar low.[9]

Other leading authors, like Dr. JoAnn Manson, gave many talks and interviews about the study following its publication. In 2023, when asked directly about the controversial findings, she claimed "it approached" nominal statistical significance. If I ever claimed an association in my research because something "approached" significance, it would be rejected on the spot.

I reached out to Dr. Manson and spoke with her for more than an hour by Zoom. I found her to be very friendly and quite charming. In our conversation she referred several times to the "increased risk of breast cancer," balancing it with other benefits of HRT.

I challenged her statement that HRT causes breast cancer and pulled up the exact numbers and odds ratios from her 2002 publication. I asked her to show me where the increase in breast cancer was found to be significant. "I completely agree with you that there is some concern that the sequentially monitored confidence interval wasn't the focus," she told me.[10] It wasn't clear to me if she was officially reversing her position that HRT causes breast cancer, so I again displayed the results from her publication and asked her if she'd like to go on the record to say that the study did not show that

HRT increased breast cancer. "The finding is very borderline," she said. I moved on to ask her about the Chicago meeting of the study authors. "It's a super sensitive topic. It's like one of the bleakest times of my life, thinking about that meeting," she replied. She didn't elaborate.

In the year following the WHI publication, some of the lead authors claimed credit for the decrease in U.S. breast cancer rates. But a closer look revealed that the decline had begun in 1999, three years before the WHI publication. Actually, rates of breast cancer went up by 0.5% annually after the 2002 publication, the year that HRT use plummeted. Regardless, Drs. Chlebowski and Anderson have claimed credit for preventing over 100,000 diagnoses of breast cancer.

Dr. Sarrel

To get the real story on HRT, I reached out to Dr. Philip Sarrel, a leading expert on estrogen. An emeritus professor of obstetrics and gynecology and of psychiatry at Yale, he graciously gave me hours of his time. He told me that he had been invited to be one of the WHI study's investigators when it was being organized, but after examining the study design and seeing several red flags, he had declined to participate in protest. He had also been amazed by how little the cardiologist leading the study had appeared to know about the field of reproductive biology.

Dr. Sarrel explained all the medical nuances on the topic. A true scientist at heart, he described how estradiol (the body's natural form of estrogen) is "oxidized" to produce nitric oxide, a molecule that dilates blood vessels, keeps them healthy and elastic, and prevents heart disease. As early as the 1890s, doctors noticed that women who had their ovaries removed developed early heart disease. Then in 1953, researchers from the Mayo Clinic studied young women who had their ovaries removed in their 20s. They all went on to develop early heart disease, including one woman who died of a heart attack at age 28.[11] In that study, among women under age 60, the average time from removing ovaries to death was 11 years. The Mayo Clinic researchers challenged the medical establishment at the time by suggesting that hormones are not just for reproduction, they also affect blood vessel health and thus, overall health.

Hormones may also be good for neurons. I was fascinated when Dr. Sarrel explained how some research on estrogen comes from the octopus, an emotionally intelligent animal that thrives on estrogen. After about a year or two of life, its estrogen levels drop precipitously, it stops eating, and it dies. What's also amazing about the octopus is that its estrogen-rich body is majestically coordinated and smart. Its eight arms can perform separate tasks independently. It can navigate mazes, solve math problems, remember, and predict. It can even use tools and take apart just about anything from a crab shell to a lock.[12] Its estradiol is believed to optimize its body's many neurons.

In the end, Dr. Sarrel concluded that the WHI cardiologists didn't understand hormones but they "made the loudest noise, so they got their message through." He has since committed his life to explaining the real science of HRT and its many benefits.

Doctors Who Refuse to Prescribe HRT

I began asking doctors who treat menopausal symptoms if they offer HRT to their patients. The prescription is simple: estrogen + progesterone if a woman still has a uterus, or estrogen alone if a woman had her uterus removed. (The progesterone helps protect the endometrial lining of the uterus and prevent uterine cancer.) Remarkably, most doctors told me they tried not to prescribe HRT because they worried about the risk of breast cancer. Some would prescribe it but only if the menopausal symptoms were extreme. Even then they would reluctantly prescribe "as little as possible for as short of time as possible," hoping the whiff of estrogen wouldn't trigger breast cancer. This, even though no randomized trial or credible study has ever shown that HRT increases a woman's risk of dying of breast cancer.

Yet to this day, the dogma lives on.

I reached out to Dr. Bill Queale, a Maryland primary care doctor that I trust. I like him because he reads everything. It turns out he is in the minority of physicians who know the truth about the faulty HRT data. "Marty, the estrogen-causes-breast-cancer idea was beaten into us so bad, it scared the crap out of most of us," he said. He estimated that a majority of the doctors in his field nationally still hesitate to prescribe it for that reason.

Perplexed as to how many doctors have been persuaded by the unsupported claims of the WHI lead authors, I began to ask women experiencing menopausal symptoms what they were being told by their doctors about their symptoms. Most were never offered HRT, or even told about the option. A few others had told me they heard it can cause breast cancer. I pointed out to them that when I recently spoke to Dr. Rossouw, the head of the WHI study, he admitted to me that the breast cancer risk was not statistically significant and that HRT was "a reasonable treatment for younger women."

In many of my discussions about the data, it struck me that the *fear* of HRT-induced breast cancer was not a scientific discussion. It's become a belief system.

Doctors who really want to believe HRT causes breast cancer will sometimes cite poorly designed studies, like the so-called "million women study." This study sounds like a clinical trial that had a million people in it, but it didn't. Instead, it was a questionnaire sent to a million women. Most women never even responded. It was also mailed to women after they had a mammogram (presumably some had the mammogram because of a suspicious lump or other concern) so it surveyed a skewed, nonrepresentative sampling of women. Others who insist HRT causes breast cancer will sometimes point to follow-up studies reported by WHI researchers. But after women were unblinded in the original study, and those on HRT were told they had a higher breast cancer risk, some religiously began an aggressive hunt for breast cancer, even if it was indolent. Other flaws in the follow-up studies have been documented in the medical literature.

As time has passed since the original WHI study, critics have pointed out even more flaws in its design and execution. For example, the study used horse urine estrogen and synthetic progesterone, not the bioidentical forms commonly used today.

In looking at the total body of medical research on the topic, the data are overwhelming. In analyzing 30 trials with a total of 26,708 women participants, HRT was not associated with an increase in cancer mortality, according to a study by researchers from Santa Clara Medical Center, Stanford, and the University of California San Francisco. Conversely, women who took HRT lived longer. In the subset of 17 trials in which women began HRT before age 60, "HRT was associated with a reduction in total mortality of 39%."[13]

The data are clear. HRT saves lives.

A Humbling Day

Sometimes patients walk into clinic with a real medical mystery. One of the most humbling cases I saw as a student was that of a 52-year-old woman that came to the surgery clinic with a three-year history of new-onset abdominal discomfort, palpitations, depression, and numbness and tingling. We doctors huddled to try to crack the case.

One doctor rattled off the need for a CT scan, a cardiac stress test, and a litany of blood tests. Another doctor wanted to do nothing because the patient had dismissed her symptoms as mild. A third doctor, always worried about malpractice liability, insisted that we get a consultation from a cardiologist, psychiatrist, neurologist, and sleep medicine specialist. He enthusiastically offered to make the referrals himself because he knew good people in each field. Incidentally, all three doctors were male.

Then, finally, a female medical student cut through the chatter and solved the enigma by interjecting two words: "It's menopause."

What? I thought. *Really?*

We had spent fewer than 15 minutes talking about menopause in medical school. I know because a female classmate, Jennifer Rosen, had complained about how the curriculum virtually skipped over the topic, as most of the rest of the class (mostly male) rolled their eyes. Could it really account for all these symptoms, some of which were severe?

Menopausal symptoms, we were told — by male professors — were merely mild hot flashes and night sweats, affecting just some women, and lasted about two years. But in fact menopausal symptoms affect 80% of women, can be severe, and last an average of 7.5 years.[14]

The patient was sent back to her primary care doctor, who cured all her symptoms with estrogen and progestin. She came back to the clinic just to tell us how much better she felt and to thank us. She had been relieved of her debilitating medical problems.

I was blown away.

Dr. Sarrel explained to me that "because of the WHI, there was little medical education about menopause. Because WHI suggested there was no safe treatment for it." That may explain why only 20% of OB/GYN residents surveyed some ten years later reported being taught about menopause in their training.[15]

Sadly, medical school education is slow to change. That's because the curriculum of every U.S. medical school is controlled by a private company that has a monopoly on accrediting medical schools and writing examinations. It's called the Association of American Medical Colleges (a company discovered to have given $500,000 to a dark money group in 2018.)[16] Because American medical education is controlled by a slow, political, distracted, and centralized authority, medical schools propagate outdated groupthink. It's not like college education, where each university can rapidly add new courses and adapt existing curricula to new scientific thinking.

A Closer Look

I saw how quickly HRT treated the immediate symptoms of menopause right before my eyes. It was one of the most vivid and rewarding fixes I had seen in medicine, the type of stuff that makes us look good as doctors. The power of HRT to alleviate the symptoms of menopause has never been controversial. But what about its long-term benefits? In reviewing the literature and talking to colleagues, I learned something amazing. There are vast and well-established benefits for a woman who starts taking HRT within ten years of experiencing menopause. HRT reduces the risk of a host of medical problems.

Let's briefly explore some of the big ones. As you will see in the next few pages, *even if* the WHI would have shown that HRT increases the risk of breast cancer, the long-term health benefits of HRT are so profound that they would far outweigh that increased risk.

Reduces Cognitive Decline (Better than Billion-Dollar Drugs)

Women taking estrogen have a 35% lower incidence of Alzheimer's. That's according to a University of Southern California study of more than 8,800 women. "Estrogen replacement therapy may be useful for preventing or delaying the onset of Alzheimer disease in postmenopausal women," the study concluded.[17]

Let's put this benefit in context. For every woman diagnosed today with breast cancer, two are diagnosed with Alzheimer's. Keep in mind that breast cancer is 90% curable. Alzheimer's has a 0% cure rate.

Researchers have long noted an association between hormones and cognition. A 2009 Mayo Clinic study of women who had both ovaries removed before menopause — thereby cutting off their hormone production — found they had an increased risk of depression and anxiety, dementia, and Parkinson-like symptoms.[18]

Other studies have identified a potential mechanism of action: Estrogen supports neuron development and maintenance throughout life.[19] More recently, a 2023 UK study of 1,178 postmenopausal women found that women who took HRT had improved memory.[20]

Danish researchers randomized 343 women in early menopause to receive HRT versus placebo and followed them for up to 15 years. They found that taking HRT for even just two to three years reduced the risk of cognitive impairment by 64%.[21] Wow.

Compare that to the hot new Alzheimer's drug, Leqembi, approved by the FDA in 2023. Leqembi was reported to slow cognitive decline in women by 12% — at an annual cost of $26,500.[22,23]

But unlike HRT, the new Alzheimer's drugs have major risks (a 13% risk of brain swelling and a 17% risk of brain bleeding), which is why there is a black-box warning on the drug's label. Those are not trade-offs I would have ever recommended for my aunt Aida, who succumbed to the cruel disease. HRT is a thousand times safer and a fortieth of the cost. I do sometimes wonder if, had my aunt taken HRT, her cognitive decline could have been prevented or delayed.

As an aside, I decided to read the entire 2023 *New England Journal* study that led to Leqembi's FDA approval. I discovered that the reported 12% reduction in Alzheimer's progression in women was *not* statistically significant (*déjà vu* of the WHI study). The results for women — who make up two thirds of the people with Alzheimer's — did not appear anywhere in the printed article, which was funded by the drug's manufacturers. I found them deep in the study's supplemental material online.

It is strange to me that America will spend billions on a drug to treat Alzheimer's, but pennies to study what actually prevents it.

Less Likely to Break a Bone from a Fall or Car Accident

Falling down is a common cause of death. Sure, the death certificate will often cite some other cause like pneumonia, but after age 65, a fall often triggers a cascade of events that can be lethal. It can be a wrist fracture causing loss of independence or an ankle or hip fracture causing immobility. In fact, the one-year mortality following a hip fracture is 22%.[24]

Remarkably, HRT lowers the risk of a fracture by 50 to 60% according to a randomized trial published in the *New England Journal.*[25] There are not a lot of ways a woman can increase her bone density and reduce her risk of a hip fracture, but HRT is one. In fact, without HRT, it doesn't matter how much calcium and vitamin D a postmenopausal woman takes for the strength of her bones. HRT helps make bones stronger.

Another study that tracked nearly 3,000 women for decades found that postmenopausal women who had taken estrogen had a 35% lower risk of hip fracture.[26] This reduced risk is especially beneficial for older women. Among women aged 80 and older, 1 in 3 will have a hip fracture as a result of osteoporosis.[27]

These benefits of HRT were known to doctors before the WHI report was released in 2002. In 1984, the NIH convened a Consensus Development Conference on Osteoporosis that met for two days of presentations by experts. The panel concluded by making strategy recommendations for addressing osteoporosis, listing first among them "ensuring estrogen replacement in postmenopausal women."[28]

Bone fractures kill women. To put this risk in context, the number of women who die each year from a hip fracture (about 40,000) is roughly equal to the number of women who die from breast cancer. As I write this book, my mom just had a close call. She fell while walking and fractured two bones, requiring surgery. Mom experienced menopause just as the WHI study came out in 2002. Her doctors never suggested HRT to her. I can't help but wonder this week if her pain, surgery, medical bills, and temporary disability could have been avoided had she been on HRT.

Prevents Heart Attacks

Heart disease is the leading cause of death in American women. HRT reduces that risk by about 50%.

What? you're probably asking. Honestly, I was shocked too. I didn't even know it was that high because we hardly ever talk about it in the medical community. I've heard a million talks and public health campaigns demonizing saturated fat, extolling CPR, and advocating putting a defibrillator in every mall in America, yet I've *never* heard one about HRT. But the data are abundantly clear.

Researchers from the University of California San Diego and Johns Hopkins did a thorough review of the research literature and concluded that most studies of HRT "show around a 50% reduction in risk of a coronary event in women using unopposed oral estrogen."[29] By comparison, statins — which are currently used by 40 million Americans — lower the incidence of heart attacks by 25 to 35%.[30]

Another study, published two years before the WHI study, looked at 70,000 postmenopausal women over 20 years and found that

HRT reduced the risk for major coronary events by almost 40%.[31] What other intervention reduces the risk of the number one cause of death in women by that much?

Another powerful observation is that women who stop taking HRT have a 26% increased risk of a fatal heart attack in the first year after stopping HRT, according to a large Finnish study.[32]

Furthermore, in 2012 Danish researchers published the results of a ten-year randomized controlled trial in over a thousand women who had recently experienced menopause. They found that HRT reduced the risk of heart attacks and other major heart problems by 52%. The authors also pointed out that prolonged use of HRT did not increase the risk of breast cancer or stroke.[33] Finally, a 2015 review of the entire body of literature on the topic by the Cochrane Library found that women who started HRT within ten years of menopause had half the rate of "death from cardiovascular causes and non-fatal myocardial infarction" and no increased stroke risk.[34]

For the heart benefits — and nearly all health benefits, for that matter — the key is that HRT must be started around menopause (or within ten years of its onset). That's when a woman's level of estrogen naturally drops and her blood vessels begin to gradually narrow and harden, a process fostered by lower levels of nitric oxide and by normal aging. The narrowing and hardening over the first ten years after menopause may be irreversible. This explains why the WHI study did not show the better cardiac outcomes seen in other studies. WHI participants started HRT at an average age of 63. That's too late.

HRT, started around the menopausal years, helps keep the walls of blood vessels soft and dilated. A consistent finding by experts I trust is that it's ill-advised to start HRT more than ten years after menopause. For women who can start HRT within ten years of menopause, those same experts will often keep women on it for life, if no complications or risk factors develop.

Reduces Colon Cancer Risk

When I've had to break the bad news to women that they have colon cancer, it sometimes leads to a long conversation with them about its causes. Some have asked if there was anything they could have done differently in their life to have prevented it. My standard answer has been no, nothing. But in 2009, three big studies reported that HRT can reduce the risk of colon cancer.

The first study looked at 56,000 women over two decades. Researchers from the University of Minnesota and the NIH found that the women who took HRT had a 25 to 45% decreased risk of colon cancer, depending on the type and duration of HRT used.[35] Another study, by the American Cancer Society, analyzing 67,000 women, found that HRT use was associated with a 24% decreased risk of colorectal cancer.[36] Finally, the *Journal of Clinical Oncology* reported in a study of more than 2,600 Israeli women that HRT was associated with a 63% reduction in the risk of colorectal cancer in postmenopausal women.[37] The microbiome, the bacterial layer that lines the gut, may also play a role, a topic we'll explore in the next chapter.

OTHER SURPRISING BENEFITS

One reason couples stop having sex when a woman goes through menopause is because of vaginal dryness, making sex painful for some women. Estrogen reduces vaginal dryness. Incidentally, women also report that HRT alleviates the dryness they notice in their nose, mouth, eyes, and scalp. Doctors tell me they have saved marriages by prescribing HRT to women. "The mental health improvement is palpable," one of them told me.

HRT may also help prevent diabetes. WHI researchers, with all their skepticism about HRT, reported in 2004 that women on HRT had a 21% lower risk of diabetes.[38] One possible mechanism for the reduction in diabetes is that women on HRT feel better, may be more active, and thus have less of the weight gain typically seen with menopause. That could be why a systematic review published in 2017 found that HRT delays the onset of Type 2 diabetes.[39,40] While the data are considered less definitive than for the other benefits of HRT, the potential implications are significant. One in seven U.S. women has diabetes.[41,42]

Finally, because HRT helps with bone density, there is also a dental benefit. A 2017 study found that severe gum disease was 44% lower in women who were taking HRT.[43] Another study by South Korean researchers found that postmenopausal women had a higher risk of gum disease, and that HRT could reduce its incidence.[44] Yet another little-known health benefit of HRT.

Overall, HRT may do more to improve the health of women over age 50 on a population level than any other medication in history.

A Few Notable Exceptions

While HRT has a long list of dramatic short-term and long-term health benefits, it is not for everyone. Some oral forms of estrogen have been suggested to slightly increase the risk of a blood clot. But this is not the case for transdermal estrogen. The very low risk of a blood clot is akin to that of oral contraceptive pills. Women with risk factors for developing a blood clot may be advised against the oral form.

For some women with endometriosis, estrogen can make it worse. Furthermore, some women who take HRT may not tolerate it because it can cause a resumption of bleeding or irritability and moodiness. Not everyone does well with it. Also, as above, no one recommends starting HRT more than ten years after menopause. Women should also be aware that the type and quality of estrogen and progesterone matter. There are "pill mills" carrying HRT made with poor quality control. Some clinics say they only offer surgically implanted pellets for HRT when women should really be offered all options, including topical, oral, and implantable.

For these and other reasons, the recommendation to take HRT should be nuanced, rather than a one-size-fits-all recommendation. Nevertheless, the vast majority of women in the world benefit from HRT when started in the first ten years after menopause.

Lowering Drug Costs

As I write this book, the FDA just approved the first medication to treat hot flashes, Veozah.[45] Already I'm noticing a barrage of Veozah ads on TV. While the ads do not have the standard people dancing and singing, Veozah does market itself as hormone-free. The obvious question that comes to my mind: Why would a healthy woman take this new medication to treat one menopausal symptom when she could take HRT to treat the same symptom and get the full spectrum of short- and long-term health benefits?

For a woman who can't take HRT, such as someone with a predisposition to blood clots or someone with active breast cancer, Veozah seems like a great medication. But otherwise, it makes no sense to me. Plus, it's much more expensive than HRT. A one-year supply of Veozah costs $7,386 at my local Costco.

As politicians scratch their heads trying to figure out how to lower drug costs in the U.S., here's a simple idea: The best way to lower drug costs in the U.S. is to stop encouraging patients to take expensive drugs when there are less expensive alternatives.

Drs. Avrum Bluming, Carol Tavris, Phil Sarrel, and others have dedicated their lives to educating doctors about the truth about HRT. Dr. Sarrel is among a group of experts from around the country who now run a foundation to educate women and physicians about the best data on the topic.[46] Visana is another group helping women navigate the healthcare system to find good care.

The leaders of the WHI have done tremendous damage to public health. Dr. Sarrel and a team of researchers published a study that estimated that up to 91,000 women have died prematurely from HRT avoidance in the first decade after the infamous WHI press conference. Dr. Sarrel told me that in the last ten years, there have been at least another 50,000 premature deaths due to the misinformation put forth by WHI leaders.[47] Looking back, telling women to avoid HRT because it causes breast cancer may have been the biggest error in modern medicine.

Women deserve an apology.

Yet, inexplicably, the dogma is still alive and well. This year, the U.S. Preventive Services Task Force, an influential board of doctors in America, renewed its guidance to avoid HRT to prevent chronic conditions because of the risk of breast cancer. The

Task Force's statement read, "The USPSTF recommends against the use of combined estrogen and progestin for the primary prevention of chronic conditions in postmenopausal persons." In response, strong articles by Dr. Langer and others pointed out the fallacy of the recommendation and urged them to take a hard look at the evidence.[48,49]

Today

Lead author Dr. Jacques Rossouw went on to be named one of *Time* magazine's hundred most influential people in 2006.[50] *Time* wrote that he and others "deserve a round of applause for their role in the WHI's mythbusting operation." As of my submitting this book manuscript, Dr. Rossouw, at age 81, is still a volunteer scientist at the NIH.[51]

I asked Dr. Rossouw if he had any regrets. He reaffirmed that he believes that HRT causes breast cancer. He did add that he wishes he would have stated "more loudly" in his press release that HRT is "a reasonable treatment for younger women" to treat menopausal symptoms. "I made sure to tell women that the absolute risks are small . . . may be less than one in a thousand . . . That didn't get picked up. You know how the media operates, they want bad news."

Dr. JoAnn Manson, another lead author

of the WHI, went on to be promoted and is now the chief of Preventive Medicine at Brigham and Women's Hospital and a professor of epidemiology at the Harvard T. H. Chan School of Public Health. She is celebrated as the fifth most cited researcher in medicine.[52]

To her credit, Dr. Manson has walked back some claims made by WHI investigators and has been open to discussing the study with critics.[53] In 2016 she admitted in an article in the *New England Journal* that "reluctance to treat menopausal symptoms has derailed and fragmented the clinical care of midlife women, creating a large and unnecessary burden of suffering."

In a 2023 interview with Dr. Manson, Dr. Peter Attia remained polite while pressing her, but he concluded the interview by telling her, "I still remain somewhat sad, because I think there's a lost generation of women. There's 20 years of women that entered menopause who were denied HRT due to the ignorance of their physicians and the irresponsibility of the media. And I look at women like my mother and mother-in-law who were entering menopause just as the WHI was coming to its conclusion, who suffered unnecessarily . . . How many millions suffered unnecessarily?"[54]

When I told Dr. Langer about Dr. Attia's frustration, he took it a step further. "We are about to lose the opportunity to help the next generation of women if we don't work hard to provide honest findings to women and doctors."

Dr. Garnet Anderson, the WHI study's statistician, went on to be named senior vice president and director of public health sciences at Fred Hutch, the highly regarded cancer center at the University of Washington, where she also holds an endowed chair. Her bio on the center's website boasts, "In 2002, she and her WHI colleagues reported that menopausal estrogen-plus-progestin therapy increased the risk of breast cancer . . . Subsequent analyses led by Hutch colleagues estimated these changes prevented 126,000 breast cancer diagnoses and saved approximately $35.2 billion in direct medical expenses." As I was writing this book in early 2023, I happen to notice a statement Anderson and a WHI colleague had published in the *New York Times* in response to an article by staff writer Susan Dominus. The title of Dominus's article, published on February 1, 2023, was "Women Have Been Misled About Menopause." In her response a few weeks later, Anderson shamelessly wrote, on behalf of the WHI steering committee, that the worldwide decrease in the use of HRT "undoubtedly has saved millions of lives and billions of U.S. healthcare dollars."[55] I wish that were true.

It would be good for the people involved in propagating the HRT-causes-breast-cancer absolutism to show some humility. It's not too late. But we've heard no apologies from the 40 WHI investigators, except for Dr. Robert Langer.

From time to time, a woman will ask me how she can find a good primary care physician or internist. I sometimes suggest that she start by asking candidates how they feel about treating menopausal symptoms with HRT. If the doc responds with "I don't prescribe it because I worry about the risk of breast cancer," my recommendation is clear. Keep looking.

CHAPTER 3

"No Downsides to Antibiotics"

Except carpet-bombing the microbiome

All truths are easy to understand once they are discovered; the point is to discover them.

— Galileo Galilei

One day in the hospital emergency department, I examined a teenager, Chris, who'd suffered repeated bouts of abdominal pain. He looked miserable. I introduced myself, tried to make him laugh with a Taylor Swift joke, and then, along with my medical student, examined him.

"No doctor has been able to figure out what's going on with him," his distressed mother told me. "Each time this happens, doctors just call it 'irritable bowel.' "

I smiled, knowing that's medical speak for "We have no idea."

I ran a bunch of tests on him, but they only revealed some inflammation of his intestines, the kind of unsatisfying, nonspecific thing we see all the time. I went back to the doctors' workroom and pored over Chris's medical records. I soon realized the most likely cause of his suffering: His microbiome had been assaulted.

The microbiome is one of the least understood organ systems in the body, yet it may be central to our health. It's a garden of billions of different bacteria, fungi, and other organisms in our gut that normally live in a healthy balance.[1]

Throughout his life Chris's microbiome had been repeatedly thrown out of whack. He was born by C-section, which means that his sterile gut at birth may have been seeded with bacteria from the hospital rather than with bacteria from the vaginal canal. He was not breast-fed, and that fact impacts the microbiome. He also loved junk food, I learned, further altering the bacteria in the microbiome. Then I saw in his records the biggest assault on his gut's bacteria: the dozen or so courses of antibiotics he had taken throughout his childhood.

His microbiome had been carpet-bombed.

I had a long conversation with Chris's mom about the microbiome. Antibiotics kill some types of gut bacteria and, as a result, other bacteria grow to fill the void. This throws off the natural balance, which can cause health problems. For example, antibiotics may cause inflammation by killing low-inflammatory bacteria, allowing bacteria that increase inflammation to flourish. We doctors sometimes assign the umbrella diagnosis of "bacterial overgrowth syndrome" to the problem. The modern-day tragedy is that approximately half of the antibiotics prescribed in the U.S. are unnecessary, an estimate that's been reaffirmed by several studies.[2]

It hasn't always been this way. Take ear infections, for example. Historically, before giving antibiotics doctors would carefully look in the ear to distinguish a bacterial versus a viral infection. Viral infections are far more common and do not respond to antibiotics. But today few doctors outside of the ear, nose, and throat (ENT) specialty are interested or skilled enough to make the distinction. It's easier not to look in the ear (especially with telemedicine) and instead to dole out antibiotics like candy. Many believe that telemedicine is all good. But a Johns Hopkins study my colleagues and I recently conducted found that a doctor is far more likely to prescribe an antibiotic in a telemedicine visit than in person. Many of those prescriptions are unnecessary — and the overprescribing of antibiotics is causing more harm than we may realize.

I had little to offer Chris, beyond suggesting some dietary changes. His mom confessed that she had always felt hesitant about giving him antibiotics for common colds. But doctors had told her, "There are no downsides to antibiotics."

It's a phrase I've heard over and over in my career. Unfortunately, it's not true.

What They Didn't Teach in Medical School

Antibiotics save lives. I've personally seen it happen many times. But they should not be overprescribed because they are also like TNT to the billions of gut bacteria that should live in harmony. Bacteria are generally considered to be bad (and gross), but bacteria in the microbiome live in a balance, and together they do amazing things for your health. They are involved in digestion, train the immune system, make vitamins, and produce serotonin, which affects mood. The bacteria of the microbiome live in a balance — and as a result, they keep you healthy.

Not only do antibiotics kill off parts of your microbiome, but they may also have immediate side effects.

This first became apparent to me as a resident when I prescribed a woman with a bladder infection an antibiotic called a quinolone. The patient later told me that after taking it, her Achilles tendon had ruptured. *What?* I thought. *How on earth can an antibiotic do THAT?* I went back and researched it. Sure enough, a spontaneous tear of the Achilles tendon was a well-known complication, one of the many I had underappreciated.

To learn more about the complications of antibiotics, I talked to my Johns Hopkins colleague Dr. Sara Cosgrove. She's an infectious diseases doctor who's dedicated her career to studying the harm of antibiotic overuse. Her research found that 20% of hospitalized patients treated with an antibiotic will experience an adverse effect, such as mild injury to their kidney or liver.[3] "Most doctors aren't aware that the complication rate is that high," Dr. Cosgrove told me. I certainly hadn't been. Minor adverse events don't typically come to our attention.

Given that so much antibiotic use is not medically necessary, these are often avoidable complications.

I asked Dr. Cosgrove about the latest research on how antibiotics may be affecting the microbiome. She referred me to Dr. Marty Blaser, a microbiome expert at

Rutgers University and formerly the chief of medicine at New York University Hospital. The topic was personal for Dr. Blaser. He and his wife, Dr. Maria Gloria Dominguez-Bello, a microbiologist, now realize their daughter took far too many antibiotics as a child. In retrospect, the couple felt terrible about giving her antibiotics for minor viral infections as she grew up. Even though they were doctors, they followed their pediatrician's orders. Many of the scripts were given with the false assurance that "there are no downsides." They thought they were doing the right thing. Their daughter now suffers from chronic digestive problems and irritable bowel symptoms — similar to Chris. This ordeal inspired Dr. Blaser to dedicate his career to microbiome research.

"We're poisoning the microbiome," he told me, referring to the overuse of antibiotics.

After several conversations with Dr. Blaser, I traveled to Rutgers University to spend a day with him in his lab. He shared research that showed how the microbiome is largely formed by the time a child is 3.[4,5] The problem is that by age 3, the average American child has already taken about four courses of antibiotics!

Dr. Blaser got a clue about the harmful effects of overusing antibiotics from an unexpected source: farmers. Animals raised for use as human food were frequently given antibiotics because it makes them fatter. Dr. Blaser did an experiment to replicate the effects using mice. He found that, sure enough, mice on antibiotics became fatter than those that did not get them.[6,7] He analyzed the number and diversity of the gut bacteria and saw the vivid effect of antibiotics on the microbiome. If this was happening to animals, he thought, *what are antibiotics doing to children?*

Then Dr. Blaser showed me a study that may be one of the most fascinating and important studies of the last few years.

Researchers at the Mayo Clinic followed every child born in Olmsted County, Minnesota, where the renowned hospital system is based, over an 11-year period. They compared the roughly 10,000 children who took an antibiotic in the first two years of life to approximately 4,000 children who did not. The children who took antibiotics grew up to have much higher rates of obesity, learning disabilities, asthma, and celiac disease.[8]

Here are the data. Compared to children who did not get antibiotics, the children given antibiotics in their first two years of life had a:

- 20% higher risk of obesity
- 21% higher risk of a learning disability
- 32% higher risk of ADHD
- 90% higher risk of asthma
- 289% higher risk of celiac disease

And that was just in the short term. Imagine what the long term might look like.

The study was powerful. It accounted for differences in health status and demographics between the two groups. But were antibiotics a cause? We can't say for certain, but the study also showed that the more antibiotic prescriptions a child received, the greater their risk of developing a chronic disease. Those are compelling data! It's something we call a dose-dependent relationship and suggests a cause and effect. Dr. Blaser said he and his colleagues recently repeated the analysis in a study population of a million children and got similar results.[9]

This study blew me away. *How had I not heard about these findings?* At Johns Hopkins, we talk about studies from around the world all the time. Geniuses scratch their heads as to what causes diseases like celiac. Patients with celiac ask what caused their disease, and we answer that it's not known. The strong correlation found in the Mayo

Clinic study suggests one cause may be right in front of us.

Dr. Blaser's team conducted an even more compelling follow-up lab experiment. They gave antibiotics to mice to alter their microbiome. Then they transferred a sample of the mice's antibiotic-disturbed microbiome to the guts of healthy mice. The result? The healthy mice suddenly got fat. There are two theories explaining why.[10] It may be that the altered garden of bacteria changed the way food is digested and absorbed by the body. Or it could be that the altered bacteria results in fewer gut hormones being produced — hormones such as GLP-1, which has been found to be produced by gut bacteria at low levels. Either way, the lab experiments revealed that the obesity the animals developed was not due to genes. It was due to an altered microbiome.

In another experiment, researchers transferred antibiotic-altered microbiome to the guts of sterile mice born in the lab. Not only did those recipient mice develop the digestive disease colitis, but so did their offspring.[11]

"You don't just inherit genes, you inherit your microbiome," Dr. Blaser told me.

Dr. Blaser likened the problem to global warming. The diversity of the microbiome is decreasing with each generation. This ongoing depletion may, in part, explain some food allergies. The incidence of food allergies had been creeping up for decades. That may have been due to a changing microbiome passed from generation to generation. In the case of peanut allergies, as we have seen, the problem was significantly compounded by immune sensitization from peanut avoidance.

Roughly 200 million people in the world today have a food allergy. Harvard's Dr. Talal Chatila has found that the microbiome of children with food allergies looks different than the microbiome in children without food allergies. I visited with him to learn more. He and his team have identified one bacterium in particular, called *Subdoligranulum variabile,* that is missing or depleted in children with food allergies. That bacterium may protect against food allergies, he believes. Now the team is experimenting with treating food allergies in humans using oral bacteriotherapy. Dr. Chatila is optimistic.

Other research teams are doing clinical studies to test the effectiveness of having people drink the bacteria that produce GLP-1, the active ingredient in the popular weight loss drug Ozempic.[12] Early results have demonstrated that drinking the bacteria *Akkermansia* and other bacteria can help people with diabetes better control their blood sugar, reducing their hemoglobin A1C by 0.6% — which is a significant reduction.[13]

Can Antibiotics Make Us Overweight and Sick?

There is also an epidemiological suggestion that taking antibiotics early in life may be associated with chronic diseases. Beginning in the post–World War II era, U.S. rates of chronic diseases have markedly increased, including rates of obesity, asthma, and diabetes.[14] It was striking to look at two U.S. maps that Dr. Blaser showed me from one of his publications. In his opinion, they suggest the need for further investigation. One map shows the states with the highest rates of antibiotic use, and the other shows the states with the highest rates of obesity. "They're essentially the same map," he told me. The striking parallel begs for a formal study that takes into account other factors that could influence obesity rates.

Blaser and his colleagues published these maps, but the publications went largely unnoticed. The information came out in a medical journal called *Annals of the American Thoracic Society,* the tenth most read journal in the field of pulmonology.[15] That's right, one of the most intriguing epidemiologic

Obesity Rates

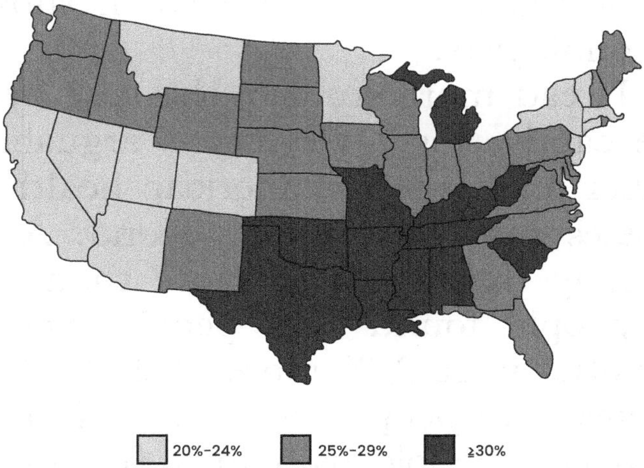

Antibiotic Prescribing*

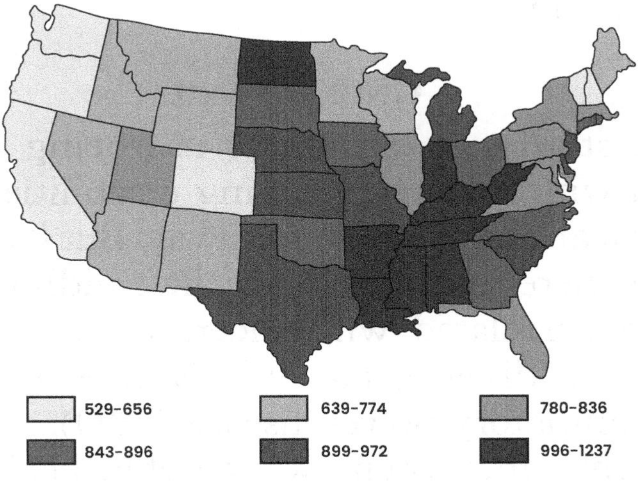

*per 1000 persons

(L. SEGAL AND M. J. BLASER, *ANNALS OF THE AMERICAN THORACIC SOCIETY*, 2014; CENTERS FOR DISEASE CONTROL AND PREVENTION, 2010) hypotheses on one of the most important health issues in America was released in a niche journal read by a small subset of pulmonologists.

As I read more studies, the case became more captivating.[16] Obesity is arguably the number one issue in American health care. Diabetes may be a close second. A Danish study that followed more than a million people found that people who took antibiotics were 21% more likely to develop diabetes than people who didn't. But here's the kicker: People who took five or more courses of antibiotics were 53% more likely to develop diabetes.[17] Again, that's a dose-dependent relationship that suggests a close association.

Uncle Nabil

The studies on antibiotic use being associated with asthma, learning disabilities, diabetes, and celiac blew me away. But it doesn't stop there. Antibiotic use in childhood has been correlated with ulcerative colitis and Crohn's disease, collectively referred to as inflammatory bowel disease (IBD).

I remember when I was a public health student at Harvard and was visiting my uncle Nabil, a busy physician in Egypt. He told me they had no Crohn's or ulcerative colitis in Egypt, an observation echoed by doctors throughout Africa and many other countries at the time. He also postulated, "In the U.S., I don't believe these diseases existed before the advent of antibiotics." Sure enough, Uncle Nabil was right.

These simple observations stuck with me as I went through residency, operating on dozens of people for ulcerative colitis and Crohn's. Incredibly, I learned about these common conditions in medical school and residency. But no one ever told us that they didn't exist before World War II, when antibiotics came on the scene, or that for several decades these diseases were limited to wealthy Western countries.

Then one day at Johns Hopkins, I heard a lecture from a visiting professor from Mount Sinai in New York, a renowned center for ulcerative colitis and Crohn's. He gave a talk about the impressive array of complex operations his center performed on these patients. It was a tour de force of technically sophisticated procedures, some performed in multiple stages over a period of months.

After his talk I asked him what caused Crohn's and ulcerative colitis.

He said we don't really know. I then asked him if it was true that in poor countries, the conditions were virtually undescribed, and that they had not been heard of before the 1940s. He agreed and appeared intrigued by the thought, but he had no comment. I didn't mean to invalidate his impressive talk with a piercing question. But at the same time, it seemed bizarre to me that the cause of these disabling diseases wasn't a part of the academic field for those specializing in it.

Within a few years of his lecture, studies began to connect antibiotic use and IBD. Children who took antibiotics were two to three times more likely to develop IBD than children who didn't.[18] As seen in the other studies, the more antibiotics a child took, the greater the risk of IBD. Then a Swedish study found that taking antibiotics in childhood was associated with a 3.5-times higher risk of Crohn's, and that the risk increased the more antibiotics the child received.[19] Another study examining the tripling of Crohn's and ulcerative colitis in Hong Kong over the past decade similarly found a marked increase in those conditions among children who took multiple courses of antibiotics.[20]

Even though these studies are not widely known, they shed light on the dogma that "there are no downsides to antibiotics."

A Global Epidemic of Dogma

The U.S. has been an outlier in the overuse of antibiotics, but poorer countries are catching up and, in many cases, far surpassing the U.S. In some countries, people take antibiotics for headaches. That's right. It makes no sense, but antibiotics are sometimes seen as a magic cure for everything. Most countries don't require a prescription — they're widely available for purchase at local pharmacies and street vendors. In some countries, parents give antibiotics to their children at the first hint of *any* health concern. This is a relatively new trend and a global health crisis in the making. A 2017 study by the World Health Organization (WHO) found that in Bangladesh and Pakistan, the average 2-year-old has already received ten courses of antibiotics![21] If the current research on microbiome damage is true, we may soon witness an explosion of chronic diseases internationally and witness a massive burden placed on global health care systems.

In fact, it's already begun.

Obesity is skyrocketing in India, China, and other countries, beginning in childhood. In fact, in urban areas of China, obesity rates among teenage boys now parallel rates in the U.S. Egypt and other countries in Africa are now dealing with a rise in chronic diseases, such as Crohn's and ulcerative colitis, that were never seen before the widespread use of antibiotics. Why? Some speculate it's the surge in processed foods and the Western diet, but that may be just one of the many "hits" to the microbiome. One thing is clear: Genes alone are not to blame. It's also well known that the Amish and Old Order Mennonite communities, in which antibiotic use is low, have extremely low rates of asthma, food allergies, and Crohn's and ulcerative colitis.

A Common Thread

As I read the various microbiome studies, it struck me that altering the microbiome may be at the root of many diseases I've been seeing throughout my career.

Take colon cancer, for example. I was taught that colon polyps — believed to be precursor to colon cancer — just happen. "We don't know what causes polyps," I told hundreds of patients who asked. But now maybe we're getting a clue. A 2017 Harvard study of more than 16,000 nurses found that nurses who took antibiotics before age 60 were more likely to have a colon polyp after age 60.[22] They also found that nurses who took an antibiotic long-term were 36 to 70% more likely to have a polyp.

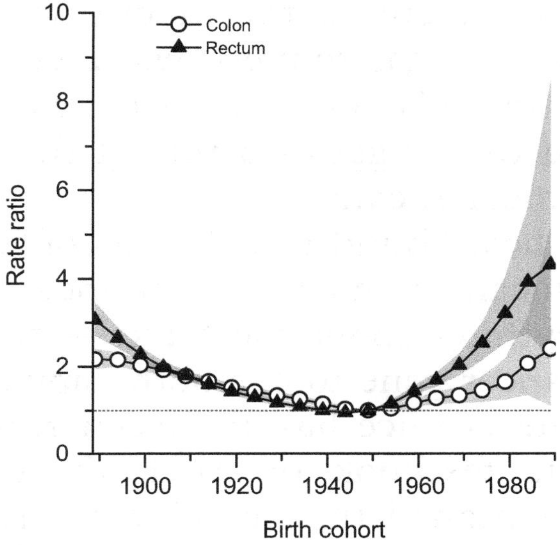

Colon cancer rates by the person's year of birth
(JOURNAL OF THE NATIONAL CANCER INSTITUTE, 2017)

Another study found that colon cancer rates correlate with a person's year of birth.[23] Look at the graph above of colorectal cancer rates in the U.S. by a person's year of birth. Colon cancer rates were steadily declining for people born before World War II, prior to the widespread use of antibiotics. But people born after 1950 have had a steady increase in colon cancer rates. We've also seen a recent rise in young people (people born in the last 50 years) getting colon cancer.

Most recently, in 2024, scientists published a study in the journal *Nature* showing that *Fusobacterium nucleatum* — a bacterium normally present in the mouth and rarely found in the gastrointestinal tract — was present in 50% of colon cancers.[24] This study further suggests a role of the microbiome in colon cancer.

I have heard hundreds of hours of teaching on colon cancer and read thousands of pages on everything about the topic — from the colon cancer gene to chemotherapy to treat it. But never once has any teacher, mentor, colleague, textbook, or article I've encountered mentioned the microbiome. It's as if it hasn't been considered "academic" to talk about it. My hope is that this book helps change that by bringing attention to the best studies on the topic.

Reverse Engineering

Breast cancer rates may also be associated with changes in the microbiome. Dr. Mary-Claire King, who discovered the BRCA genes, which convey an increased breast cancer risk, published an ominous observation in 2003. She showed that rates of breast cancer are higher for women born after 1940, compared to women born before 1940, even when the women have the same genetic predisposition.[25] Does the overuse of antibiotics play a role in rising breast cancer rates? We can't make conclusions from epidemiological data alone. But the fact that the increases seem to have the same post–World War II rise as other diseases warrants further investigation. I appreciate the need to fund research on how to treat breast cancer with chemotherapy, but we also need research dollars to study what *causes* breast cancer.

Dr. Blaser is now trying to "reverse engineer" common medical problems to look for causes and potential treatments. He's asking what diseases began to rise in the 1940s and '50s when broad antibiotic use began. In one experiment in his lab, introducing antibiotics early in the life of mice accelerated the onset of Type 1 diabetes.[26] This experiment was conducted in mice genetically predisposed to develop Type 1 diabetes. In another experiment, his team is looking to see if mice given antibiotics are more or less likely to develop Alzheimer's.[27]

It turns out a lot of medical conditions began to increase starting in the 1940s and '50s. If we study the microbiome properly, we may be able to finally crack the nut on diseases for which treatments have been stagnant for decades. Dr. Blaser told me that autism fits the pattern. Autism rates have increased steadily since the 1940s. The Mayo Clinic study, which Dr. Blaser collaborated on, has already found a link between use of one type of antibiotic, cephalosporin, and autism.[28]

In chapter 2, "OMG HRT," we discussed the important role of estrogen in the body. During my time at the Blaser lab at Rutgers, I learned that the microbiome can also affect estrogen levels.[29] Dr. Abigail Armstrong is studying this association closely and showed me impressive data confirming the interaction. It demonstrates that certain bacteria in the microbiome help break down estrogen into its active form, thus increasing levels. This is one of many new areas of research suggesting that what goes in our mouth and shapes our microbiome has broad implications for our health.

What's Altering the Microbiome?

A newborn is born sterile, that is, with no bacteria in its gut. Its microbiome is formed from vaginal bacteria the baby picks up during delivery,[30,31] along with bacteria from the mom's skin and breast milk and kisses from its mommy and daddy. By contrast, babies born by C-section, like my patient Chris, are extracted from a sterile womb into a sterile operating room, bypassing exposure to the vaginal canal as the natural first bacterial exposure.[32] As a result, their microbiome can be seeded from bacteria that normally live in the hospital. And because women who have a C-section are routinely given an antibiotic just prior to the procedure, their babies are born with antibiotics in their system. This is especially unfortunate: A study of more than 55,000 patients found that there is no difference in surgical infection rates when the antibiotics are given to a mother after her baby is born.[33]

One study found children born by C-section were up to three times more likely to develop asthma than those born vaginally.[34] And a 2023 *JAMA* study found that children born by C-section were more likely to develop colon cancer, another potential explanation for why this cancer is on the rise in young people.[35] In addition, a lack of breast-feeding has been associated with inflammatory bowel disease (IBD).

There are many things going on here that are altering the microbiome. The general rise in the use of antibiotics has corresponded with the rise in C-sections, the decline of breast-feeding, and the mainstreaming of high-sugar and ultra-processed food. That could be a quadruple threat to the microbiome.[36] Now, when I hear of a 40-year-old with colon cancer or IBD, despite having no traditional risk factors, I wonder whether they frequently took antibiotics, were born by C-section, were breast-fed, or ate a lot of unhealthy foods.

We are early in our understanding of the microbiome, and we need to be studying what other factors have an influence. For example: Does fluoride in drinking water play a role? Fluoride kills bacteria, which is exactly why people believe it prevents cavities. Do microplastics influence the microbiome? One study suggested the average person may consume up to one credit card's worth of microplastics every week.[37] How about alcohol? And what about pesticides? The average nonorganic strawberry contains 7.8 different pesticides, according to a U.S. Department of Agriculture report.[38] If those pesticides kill pests, it's possible they also kill some bacteria in the microbiome. The same could be true for weed killers used in farming, like glyphosate. If it kills weeds, what might it be doing to some bacteria in the gut? I spoke with Dr. Suchitra Hourigan, one of the few microbiome researchers at the NIH. She is currently studying how common over-the-counter medications like Pepto Bismol may be damaging the microbiome.[39]

It's time for the medical community to apply the same rigor and funding to microbiome research that it applies to studying heart disease, cancer, and other diseases. Food and chemicals that are not toxic in isolation could be changing the microbiome in ways we have not yet fully understood. They may be having a dramatic effect on our health.[40]

The microbiome factor reframes many old scientific questions. For example, for the last 60 years the question whether artificial sweeteners cause cancer has been debated. Study after study has failed to demonstrate a direct association. But maybe asking if they *cause* cancer is not the right question. Maybe we should be investigating whether they *change the microbiome*. A 2022 study[41] by researchers from Johns Hopkins, Germany, and Israel published in the journal *Cell* showed that artificial sweeteners do change the microbiome, detailing the change with each type of sweetener. The next question is: Are these changes consequential?

"There is a lot of stuff we ingest that we take for granted, that may have an effect on the microbiome. We need more research to better understand what's going on," Harvard's Dr. Chatila told me.

BACTERIOTHERAPY

Bacteriotherapy is the new science of giving patients bacteria or other molecules to help repair an altered microbiome. The most dramatic example of this approach is for *Clostridium difficile* colitis, a disease that took the life of one of my patients years ago.

A few years after her death, in 2013, researchers published an article in the *New England Journal* about a series of patients who'd been successfully treated for *C. diff* colitis by infusing small doses of liquid feces from another person into their intestine.[42] The FDA blocked it for years, but patient groups won out and sent a blunt message to government bureaucrats: Stop regulating shit. Today prescribing a pill with bacteria from the colon (i.e., stool) of healthy people is a standard treatment for patients with recurrent *C. diff* colitis. It works 99% of the time. It sounds a little gross, but given the option between major surgery and a bacteria pill, most patients prefer the latter.

Probiotics — consumable gut bacteria in liquid or pill form — are now being used to treat psychiatric illness, and they have the potential to unlock what causes mental illness. A Johns Hopkins colleague, Dr. Robert Yolken, and researchers at Sheppard Pratt Hospital recently reported that hospitalized patients with mania who were sent home with a type of probiotics were less likely to bounce back and get readmitted.[43]

Current studies are evaluating if giving gut bacteria to people with bipolar disorder will help them. Since some bacteria are known to produce serotonin and other molecules that act on the brain, it's plausible that we are on the brink of a few major breakthroughs. Most antidepressants work by increasing serotonin levels. It's entirely conceivable that bacteria could do that, or even act as a substitute.

Probiotics are very popular. Some people benefit from them, but most don't work. The market is flooded with products that have not been scientifically evaluated. Popular probiotics seem to come and go, based on which has the best marketing or what's trending on Instagram. We need more research on restoring the balance in the microbiome. We also need more research on the role of food as medicine, an often-neglected part of modern medicine's pharmacopeia. As new research elucidates which probiotics and foods can help treat disease, investors will flock to this space as they consider the mammoth potential market for probiotics to disrupt the current medication-industrial complex.

Intellectual Curiosity

As I reviewed the impressive data that ties antibiotic use in childhood to chronic diseases and even cancer, it struck me how simple the studies were to perform. It's not complicated for researchers to give mice an antibiotic and watch them get fat. A student could have done it as her seventh-grade science fair project. It shouldn't be any harder for the tens of thousands of university labs in the country. Even the epidemiological studies are fairly straightforward. Where are the National Cancer Institute, the Susan G. Komen foundation, and the dozens of major cancer centers on this research?

Chronic diseases account for 75% of our health care spending in the U.S. Our $4.5 trillion health care system is the largest industry in America, and yet it still cannot meet the need.

Many of the conditions Dr. Blaser and the Mayo Clinic researchers identified in their study to be closely associated with childhood antibiotic use — such as asthma, learning disabilities, and celiac disease — are conditions for which there has been little real scientific progress in recent decades. It's time to explore fresh ideas.

Instead, we're spending billions of dollars researching old ideas. Much of our work has hit a dead end and has not translated into meaningful improvements. It's amazing that we can spend billions treating conditions with no benefit while spending pennies to learn what causes the conditions. I sometimes wonder if the culture of medicine plays a part. Our high-volume, memorize-and-regurgitate culture of medical education seems to be stifling our intellectual curiosity.

In recent decades, we've witnessed increasing rates of ulcerative colitis, Crohn's, irritable bowel, and colon cancer in young people. It's time for the NIH to be proactive and expand its research funding priorities to support more research on the microbiome. Solid preliminary data, as laid out above, warrants a bigger research effort.

Microbiome research can be done at a fraction of the cost of drug development. This is not the Manhattan Project or the lunar landing; it's just basic research. In fact, many of the studies Dr. Blaser carried out were done by students under his direction. They are not hard to perform, but they have far-reaching implications for global health.

A Specialty with No Home

Many of the compelling studies about the microbiome that I read along this learning journey are from top scientists at leading medical centers. Yet these studies are not well known, even in the medical community.

I think that's in part because they have an identity problem. Which medical specialty should they fall under? Which specialty conference is the right one at which to present the findings? Microbiome research is foundational to the fields of gastroenterology, pediatrics, psychology, obstetrics, nutrition, public health, and infectious diseases. But it goes largely unnoticed by all of them. Published studies get lost in a sort of research Bermuda triangle.

Medical specialties can live in silos, and silos can stifle progress. From the first day in medical school, everyone continually asked me, "What specialty are you thinking of going into?" Honestly, it got annoying. I wanted to study the whole body, surgical and nonsurgical fields, and our entire medical system, but there was no residency for that. Instead, I felt like I was given a diagram of the nine organ systems and told, "Pick your favorite organ." I did (gastrointestinal surgery and surgical oncology), but then quickly returned to my first love: the entire health care system.

Microbiome research sits at the intersection of several specialties. It needs to come to the forefront of medicine. Raising money for research on bacteria in the colon is a lot harder than raising money for breast cancer.

But these are some of the biggest issues in health care today. Let me know if you see a "Race for the Microbiome" or a dance-a-thon at your local high school to raise money to fight the overuse of antibiotics.

The Next Pandemic

As I was sleeping on my office sofa, while on call at the hospital one night, I got summoned to see a 74-year-old woman in septic shock. The ICU doctors knew exactly what had made her critically ill: Her colon had been infected by the aforementioned bacteria *C. diff,* also known as *C. diff* colitis. For most of my career, we physicians cured this infection as fast as we diagnosed it, with an antibiotic. But this patient had a type of *C. diff* that was resistant to every antibiotic. As a result, the ICU doctors were helpless. All they could do was to cheer on the patient's immune system as it fought the infection. But the patient was losing the battle. In dire straits, the doctors called me as a last resort — to surgically remove her colon.

I've seen patients like this deteriorate quickly. The infection moves fast, so I mobilized my team and rushed the patient to the operating room. Over the course of the next 45 minutes, we wrestled out the left side of her large intestine. Her blood pressure was wildly unstable before and during the operation. But it suddenly became stable when we clamped each end of the infected area and cut off the infected colon's blood supply. We removed the infected colon and plopped it in a plastic bin. The patient made it back to the ICU, and we were hopeful she had a chance, but sadly the physiologic stress to her body had been too much. Her organs began to fail. She never woke up and passed away the next day. We had raced to do the operation as fast as we could, but it was too late.

Every general surgeon has a similar story from the last 10 to 15 years, because we are living in a new era: the era of antibiotic resistance. I was later told how she got the *C. diff* infection. A week prior, she had been given the antibiotic amoxicillin for a minor bruise after a fall — a bruise for which an antibiotic was not indicated. This spark ignited a forest fire. While amoxicillin pills sound innocent, they killed the "good bacteria" in her colon, allowing the *C. diff* bacteria to take over.

C. diff is the most vivid microbiome disease in medicine. Over the last 15 years, operating on a person to remove their colon because of a resistant *C. diff* infection has gone from a 1-in-a-million situation to a frequent occurrence. In recent years in the U.S., more people will die from *C. diff* than from influenza.[44] Moreover, the number is rising each year with no end in sight.

It's not just *C. diff.* Another resistant bacteria called carbapenem-resistant Enterobacteriaceae (CRE) used to be treated with the antibiotic carbapenem, considered a "drug of last resort." But now it's not working. Like *C. diff,* this type of bacteria is notorious for infecting people in the hospital. The mortality from it went from around 0% when I was a resident to 40 to 50% today.[45] Similarly, pediatricians are increasingly seeing ear infections from *Staphylococcus aureus* and other common bacteria, for which no antibiotic is effective. They have no choice but to let the child ride out the infection as they provide treatment for the pain and fever. It's getting bad. Yet this early pandemic has received little media attention.

You may be thinking: Why don't we create a new antibiotic? Well, we've been creating new antibiotics for decades, but we can't keep up.

New antibiotic development cannot keep pace with the rate of bacterial resistance. Compounding the problem: The number of new antibiotics being developed each year is dwindling because the market for them is small relative to the market for ailments like wrinkles or dry eyes.

Average time to develop resistance

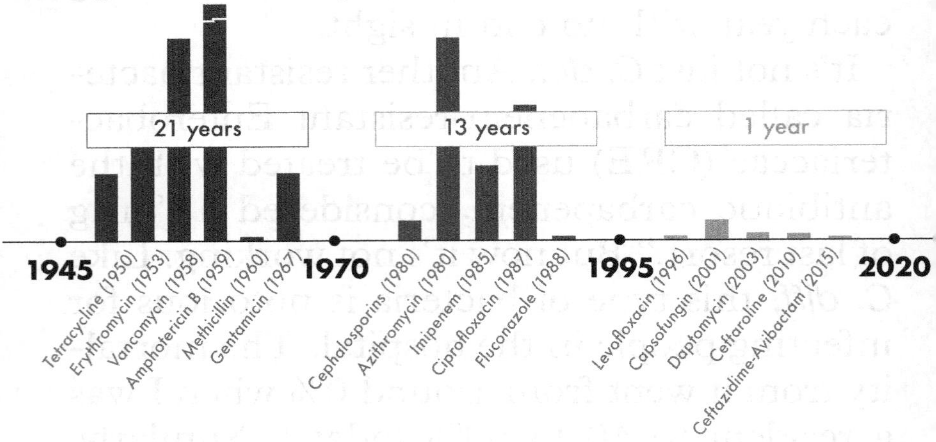

(CENTERS FOR DISEASE CONTROL AND PREVENTION, *JOURNAL OF GLOBAL HEALTH REPORTS*)

It used to take 21 years on average for bacteria to become resistant to a new antibiotic. Now it takes an average of one year. Today, the CDC lists different types of antibiotic-resistant bacteria that are circulating in the U.S. It classifies five of them as "urgent threats" to human health.[46] This is an emerging crisis. The patient I operated on was but one casualty.

The carnage of the Covid pandemic is now clear to everyone. As people try to predict the odds of a future pandemic, the reality is that the next pandemic has already begun. It's not one that rips through countries in a matter of months. It's a slower-growing pandemic, yet it is projected to kill 10 million people a year by 2050.[47]

What You Can Do

Antibiotics are not overused in humans alone. In the U.S., roughly half of antibiotics are sold to farms for raising animals in crowded conditions. And once the animals develop drug resistance to the bacteria, it can jump to humans.

In response to the antibiotic resistance problem, a few fast-food chains, such as Chipotle, have championed antibiotic-free animal products. Growing public demand for antibiotic-free foods can move markets toward better health and address the next antimicrobial-resistance pandemic. Everyone plays a critical role in preventing antimicrobial resistance, including health professionals. In the same way that we as a profession tackled smoking with a concerted educational effort, so too can we educate the public about antibiotic overuse.

We Can't Say We Weren't Warned

One day, walking into his laboratory after returning from vacation, Dr. Alexander Fleming discovered that the window in his lab had been inadvertently left open. A fungus had blown in and landed on his petri dishes where he was growing bacteria. He soon noticed that the bacteria were dead in the spots where the fungus had landed. The year was

1928, and that fungus would soon become known to the world as penicillin. It would revolutionize every field of medicine. Within a few decades, women would no longer routinely die from childbirth, children would not lose their hearing from ear infections, and surgery would be safe for the first time.

Many people know that penicillin ushered in the modern era of medicine, but what they may not know is that in 1945, as the antibiotic was beginning to be commonly used, Dr. Fleming issued an ominous warning. The "public will demand" the new miracle drug, he said, and that demand would begin "an era . . . of abuses." In an interview later that same year, he issued a stern warning: "The thoughtless person playing with penicillin treatment is morally responsible for the death of the man who succumbs to infection with the penicillin-resistant organism. I hope this evil can be averted."[48] His discovery was an accident, but his warning was deliberate.

Fleming's warning was also prophetic. The overuse of antibiotics is driving resistance and creating superbugs that are killing people. At the root of the overprescribing problem is a cavalier attitude reflected in sayings such as "Antibiotics probably won't help, but they won't hurt." It may be one of the most damaging myths of modern medicine.

It's amazing how much time we spend in medical school on memorizing and regurgitating information that we never need to know on the fly. What's lost in that rote style of education is the wisdom to know what's appropriate in medical care.

The problem of overprescribing antibiotics is getting so bad that, at many U.S. hospitals, doctors are not allowed to prescribe certain antibiotics without an infectious diseases doctor approving the request.

Antibiotics should be prescribed precisely to save a life or prevent disability. We've discussed overuse, but under-use can also be a problem. Some children are tragically *not* given antibiotics they need for severe ear infections, and as a result they can experience hearing loss and perhaps even fall behind in school because it goes unrecognized. Antibiotics can rescue a patient dying of pneumonia and they can restore sight to a person with an eye infection. But people should stop demanding antibiotics from their doctor for conditions in which they don't even work. In addition, doctors should not prescribe them just to get a five-star rating online. The modern-day consumerist culture is contributing to the epidemic. The purpose of this chapter is not to demonize antibiotics, it's to stop the overkill of prescribing them when they are not medically indicated.

The alarming current trajectory of bacterial resistance means antibiotics will become increasingly less efficient. They may even stop working, threatening to undo a century of progress in medicine. Surgery could once again become a dangerous procedure as it was in the 1800s and maternal mortality from childbirth could soar. Antibiotic stewardship is everyone's responsibility.

"No downsides"

I think about antibiotics a lot in my day-to-day life, in everything from purchasing food to caring for patients. I'm reminded of the gross overuse of antibiotics every time I see a hospital protocol prompt me to prescribe one to a patient undergoing a minor procedure who doesn't need them, just to comply with a national quality measure. I think about them every time I hear about a death from a food-borne *E. coli* bacteria outbreak in the news. I think about it every time I see people in the emergency room for irritable bowel.

The doctors and researchers currently tackling this problem give me hope. Dr. Sara Cosgrove is part of a group of doctors working tirelessly to raise awareness about the problem of antibiotic overuse. Similarly, a group of 20 biologists and anthropologists have formed a group that's working on the issue.[49] Dr. Blaser and Dr. Dominguez-Bello are actively leading more research on the microbiome, and they are traveling around the world to raise awareness.

Antibiotics can save lives. But they won't any more at the current rate of overuse. So the next time you hear the phrase "There are no downsides to antibiotics," let people know that a mountain of evidence says otherwise.

CHAPTER 4

My Uncle Sam Loves Eggs

The truth about cholesterol

As "bandwagon" investors join any party, they create their own truth — for a while.

— Warren Buffett

Whenever I'm in South Florida, I feel great. I always leave feeling stronger and healthier. It's no wonder that all the folks I meet there seem to think they're going to live forever.

When people find out in casual conversation that I'm a doctor, they often start peppering me with questions — a part of the job that all doctors become accustomed to. That was the case when I met an older lady named Betty, who asked me to explain what causes cancer.

I gave her a generic answer. But she persisted, sharing how her friend had recently died of pancreatic cancer.

"It's so tragic, she died in her sleep," she said, perplexed. "It just came out of the blue. I was *just* having lunch with her a few months ago and *boom*. And just like that, she's gone! Doc, how can that possibly happen?"

I decided to engage with her and delicately asked, "How old was your friend?"

"One hundred and three," she replied.

What? Umm . . . okay. Yes, it's tragic, I agree, but making it to 103 is a win.

How long do these Florida people expect to live? I wondered.

Another guy I met on the golf course told me he had just hit 100 years old. I asked him for his reflections on life.

"The first fifty were the hardest," he quipped.

When I asked for his secret to long life, he replied, "Staying active and feeling young."

Then it hit me. Florida's high density of hair specialists, beauty salons, coconut oil, fresh fruit, dermatologists, yoga classes, and sunshine makes people feel young, like they're going to live forever.

But my uncle Sam has his own secret to a happy South Florida life . . .

The Happiest Man Alive

Uncle Sam is one of the biggest beneficiaries of the Florida sun. At age 93, he swims, cooks, and hugs his family every day. To give you a visual, Uncle Sam is a tall Egyptian man with mocha skin, the strength of an ox, and a friendly demeanor. He's gifted with a dimple in each cheek and has a smile so powerful it gets him free food at Chick-fil-A. Everyone in the family speculates that he probably even sleeps with a big smile on his face.

Put simply, he's the happiest man alive.

And one of the daily routines that makes Uncle Sam so happy is eating eggs.

Each day, after swimming, he goes up to his apartment and prepares eggs the way his parents did when he was growing up in Egypt. He scrambles them with whole milk to add a little fluffiness and seasons them with cumin, salt, and pepper; and he likes to eat them with tomato, cheese, and fresh bread. He's eaten two eggs this way almost every morning since he was a boy. It's always been his happy place.

But Uncle Sam's eggs routine came to a screeching halt when he immigrated to the U.S. in the 1970s. He came with his wife and kids to flee a tide of communism and to seek a new life. Once he completed the move, he walked in to see his first American doctor for a checkup.

The doctor performed a routine physical and ran some basic labs. Based on Uncle Sam's borderline-high level of cholesterol (not unusual for people of Mediterranean descent) and the inventory the doctor had taken of his diet, the doctor issued a stern warning.

"No more eggs. Eggs have a lot of cholesterol."

Uncle Sam was devastated, but he had heard that American doctors were the best in the world, so he reluctantly cut back on eggs. It was hard. At times, he pondered what was worse: his new life without eggs, or communism? With every subsequent doctor visit, the conversation began with "How are you doing with the eggs?" as if he were a heroin addict. Each time, my overly honest uncle would embarrassingly admit that he was sneaking some eggs, only to be schooled on how it was directly resulting in cholesterol depositing in his arteries and clogging them up. "Each plate of eggs is going to shorten your life a wee bit," the doctor scolded him.

After a few years of battling eggs, the doctor's fixation on them ended with a truce. If Uncle Sam agreed to limit his egg consumption to once a week, the doctor would allow him to eat egg whites only (never mind that the yolk was Uncle Sam's favorite). But after a few months of reluctantly getting teased with the delicious taste of eggs, Uncle Sam surrendered. "My kids were growing up and I wanted to live long, so I decided to go all-in and eliminate eggs altogether," he recalled. He believed this sacrifice would allow him to spend more days on this earth.

Per his doctor's orders, Uncle Sam had also switched to eating low-fat foods. He switched from butter to margarine. (For younger readers, margarine is a food that humans ate in the last century perceiving it to be healthy despite it being comprised of processed vegetable oils, including corn, cottonseed, canola, safflower, soy, and sunflower, with trace pesticides mixed with hydrogenated fats and other assorted molecules that do not appear in nature.) Uncle Sam complained that American (no-fat) milk tasted like water. He missed the flavor of natural fats in the foods he loved to cook. He was told to read food labels when shopping, to look for cholesterol and avoid it. He gave up lobster because his doctor told him it was high in cholesterol. All in all, he and his doctor spent an inordinate amount of time on the topic. During those difficult years, Uncle Sam was still smiling, but he was wistful. We all could see he yearned for his daily eggs.

Watching his dad avoid his favorite foods for decade after decade wore the most on his son, my cousin Morris. He became a gastroenterologist and eventually researched the topic extensively. Morris learned the real story behind the demonization of cholesterol and saturated fat: The "evidence" that it caused heart disease was shoddy at best. He encouraged his dad to eat butter, whole milk, and the eggs he treasured. After years of discussion, Morris finally convinced him.

"It took me thirty years to undo the dogma the doctor ingrained in my dad," Morris told me. "The doctors had scared him to death!"

Thankfully, Morris was able to end his dad's miserable 30-year egg abstinence. Today, in his tenth decade of life, Uncle Sam is eating eggs again. He's back to being the happiest man alive.

The Dietary Cholesterol Myth

One of the most common recommendations of modern medicine has been for people to avoid cholesterol. It's been foundational to public health and helped shape the modern food industry. The concept sounds logical and has had a broad chorus of expert support, including from large physician associations. They believed they had the antidote to fight heart disease, America's number one cause of death, and were busy saving lives with their message that cholesterol avoidance saved lives.

There was just one problem: It was never true.

Study after study has failed to demonstrate the connection between dietary cholesterol and heart disease, or between the cholesterol in your diet and the cholesterol levels in your blood. To the contrary, strong scientific research has revealed a stark reality: The cholesterol you eat is generally not absorbed by the body. That's because the vast majority of cholesterol in food has a bulky side-chain molecule connected to it that does not allow it to be absorbed. (In scientific terms, dietary cholesterol is esterified.)

Dietary cholesterol comprises a small fraction of the human body's cholesterol. The vast majority of cholesterol in the body is made by the body. In fact, every cell in your body makes cholesterol. Moreover, cholesterol is not bad. In fact, every cell in the body has a wall that is made out of cholesterol. Cholesterol is also the building-block precursor for estrogen, progesterone, testosterone, and corticosteroids — critical hormones for normal physiology and health.

A 2018 study by Dr. Ghada Soliman of City University of New York reviewed dozens of studies on the topic and concluded, "Extensive research did not show evidence to support a role of dietary cholesterol in the development of CVD [cardiovascular disease]."[1] That's exactly why the government's dietary guidelines recently dropped dietary cholesterol limits.[2]

I couldn't help but notice that Dr. Soliman's study commented on eggs in particular. "Considering that eggs are affordable and nutrient-dense food items, containing high-quality protein . . . it would be worthwhile to include eggs in moderation as a part of a healthy eating pattern." Amazing. It's as if the study had been written for Uncle Sam!

In a 2020 study that also evaluated eggs, an international team of researchers looked at 177,000 people and found that higher egg intake (seven or more eggs per week compared with less than one egg per week) was not associated with an increase in one's blood cholesterol levels, cardiovascular disease, or mortality.[3] Another win for Uncle Sam.

Finally, while there are many health benefits to exercise, exercise does not lower one's cholesterol. Yet this has been the logic offered to the public by the medical establishment for decades.

The fact that dietary cholesterol plays almost no role in blood cholesterol has actually been known since the 1950s. And more recently, in an uncharacteristic act of humility, the American Heart Association (AHA) acknowledged this fact in 2015, albeit quietly. But for the prior half century, the AHA and the broader medical establishment locked arms and walked off a cliff together. Some critics have alleged that this may have been fostered by dollars flowing from pharmaceutical companies that make cholesterol-lowering drugs to the association and individual researchers in the field. Regardless of whether pharma played a role, this mob mentality beat up on cholesterol and saturated fat so much that any challengers to the dogma were dismissed as heretics.

A few doctors were courageous enough to ask questions.

Groupthink on Cholesterol

This story may change the way you look at every meal, shop at the grocery store, and cook. It's the true story of how the medical establishment rallied together to advance the leading medical recommendation handed down to the public for most of the last 70 years, a recommendation that governed every encounter with an overweight person and continues to loom large to this day.

Prior to the 1900s, heart attacks were rare, and were hardly described in the medical literature. But in the early 1900s, heart attacks steadily increased in prevalence, and by 1921 they emerged as the number one cause of death in the U.S., surpassing infection.[4] Then on September 24, 1955, President Dwight D. Eisenhower had a heart attack. Fearful that heart attacks could strike anyone at random like lightning, a panicked public demanded to know what caused them.

Dr. Ancel Keys, a non-physician physiologist from the University of Minnesota, rose to answer the question. It was from eating fat, he claimed. Dr. Keys came up with the idea when he was visiting Naples, Italy, and was told that heart attack rates were lower there than in the U.S. He attributed the lower rate to the Italians eating less animal fat than Americans. His hypothesis proposed that eating saturated fat increased cholesterol, which in turn increased the risk of heart attacks.

But fat and cholesterol are different. They are different molecules, and each has an entirely different physiology in the body. Keys suspected that eating high-cholesterol foods had no effect on heart disease. He had tried feeding research subjects high-cholesterol foods and found that it didn't budge their blood cholesterol levels. In fact, as far back as 1954, he admitted that "the evidence — both from experiments and from field surveys — indicates that cholesterol content, per se, of all natural diets has no significant effect on either the cholesterol level or the development of atherosclerosis in man."[5] So he had turned his attention to vilifying saturated fat.

As to what caused Eisenhower's heart attack, there were other theories held by experts at the time, but Dr. Keys was a handsome, persuasive man as well as politically connected. He had the ear of Harvard's Dr. Dudley White, Eisenhower's personal physician. So Dr. White blamed the president's heart attack on eating fat and switched the president to a strict low-cholesterol, low-fat diet.[6]

In the three years following Eisenhower's heart attack, Keys seized the momentum to take his theory to the public stage. He whipped out 20 articles on the topic and tried to cement his theory by conducting a study of several countries. The results of his study were depicted in a famous graphic, depicting a direct association between fat and heart disease.[7]

"It must be concluded that dietary fat somehow is associated with cardiac diseases mortality, at least in middle age," Dr. Keys boldly declared.

Dr. Keys, who had connections in Europe,

presented his preliminary data to the WHO in 1955.[8] But there he got torn to pieces. Doctors in the audience pointed out that the countries in his study seemed cherry-picked, that many were coastal countries, and that his sampling method was grossly inadequate.

But the U.S. medical community applauded and the media trumpeted his findings. *Time* magazine put him on the cover.[9]

Initially, the AHA did not support his theory. Their experts had been reluctant to give medical advice on the issue, citing a lack of scientific evidence. But Dr. Keys was a slick and aggressive politician. He leveraged his friendship with Dr. White, who was also a founder of the AHA, and got himself appointed to a key committee in the organization. On that committee he persuaded the other members and the organization's leadership to support his hypothesis.

Over the next 15 years, large clinical trial after large clinical trial was done to test Dr. Keys's ideas. None supported it. Some would show no reduction in heart disease deaths when people ate less fat or less saturated fat, and some found the low-fat diet resulted in lower heart disease deaths. None, however, showed that people actually lived longer if they applied Dr. Keys's theory. But this lack of confirmation didn't seem to matter to the AHA experts, who had been charmed by the doctor. At the same time, the sugar industry quietly paid scientists who demonized fat.[10] They funded research that downplayed the risks of sugar and highlighted the hazards of fat.[11]

In 1961, with Keys now at the helm of a key AHA committee, the organization adopted his position, telling men to avoid fat to prevent heart attacks and strokes. Women would be added later to the recommendation. Within ten years, they extended the recommendation to every human being 2 years old and up. It's worth noting that the AHA had been paid $1.7 million by Procter & Gamble, the makers of Crisco, which advertised itself as lower in fat than butter. By the 1990s, the low-fat recommendation was cemented into the government's infamous food pyramid. Soon, public health campaigns to avoid fat took off as textbooks, a series of government reports, and even CPR classes taught that fat causes heart disease.

Wait a Minute . . .

Not every doctor jumped on the fat-causes-heart-attacks bandwagon. Some notable experts argued that the Keys study was too crude and did not account for many other factors. His "Six Countries Study" (a seventh country was added later and the study was renamed the "Seven Countries Study") oddly left out countries that didn't support his theory — most notably Germany, France, and Switzerland, all countries that were known for their consumption of high-fat foods but that concurrently had a low prevalence of heart disease. In addition, Keys had only interviewed about 30 people from each of the countries included, and he'd conducted his diet survey during Lent, when people strictly avoided fat.[12] Some researchers who had objected to Keys's presentation at the WHO exposed the flaws of his study by publishing a more comprehensive analysis of the European data.[13]

Crushing Dissent

Dr. John Yudkin, a prominent British nutrition expert, challenged Dr. Keys throughout the 1960s and '70s. He argued that sugar was the leading driver of inflammation causing heart disease, not saturated fat. As early as 1957, he wrote that "both the proponents and opponents of a dietary [fat] hypothesis are quoting only those data which support their view." In his book *Pure, White, and Deadly,* Yudkin made a strong scientific rebuttal of Dr. Keys's hypothesis, but few doctors were convinced. Keys was their man.

Dr. Yudkin saw Dr. Keys's hypothesis "go viral" and watched the food industry increasingly pound sugar and salt into foods in order to make them low-fat and still retain taste. In a 1974 *Lancet* article he warned, "The cure should not be worse than the disease."[14]

But Dr. Yudkin was no match for Dr. Keys and his converts. The American doctor was building an army of supporters, many of whom were key influencers who controlled the high grounds of medicine.[15] In some instances, Dr. Keys ridiculed Dr. Yudkin in articles and speeches. Piling on, doctors with academic pageantry and the power players tied to the food industry destroyed Yudkin's reputation.[16] Gary Taubes, an independent journalist and a meticulous historian of this era (and a friend of mine), told me, "The idea that sugar could cause heart disease was viewed as quackery, and Yudkin was unable to swim against the current." Dr. Yudkin had been mocked by other doctors so much, his career would never recover, and that was even before the era of social media and unthrottled smears on Google. Dr. Yudkin had a distinguished career at Queen Elizabeth College, where he was chair of physiology and then professor of nutrition. But eventually his lab was shut down when his department got a new boss who didn't like what Yudkin was saying.[17] His new boss was a believer in Dr. Keys's fat hypothesis.

The sugar industry was also unhappy with Dr. Yudkin's views. Concerned about the potential impact of his writings on public opinion, they sponsored the Harvard School of Public Health to write an article for the *New England Journal.* It singled out fat and cholesterol as causing heart disease and downplayed Dr. Yudkin's findings that sucrose consumption was a major risk factor.[18,19]

Dr. Keys and his allies crushed his British counterpart, but there were other medical experts, including his own colleagues at the University of Minnesota, who thought Dr. Keys could be dangerously wrong. By 1975, in an editorial in the *New England Journal,* Dr. Henry Blackburn, who worked closely with Keys at the University of Minnesota, commented on the debate. "Two strikingly polar attitudes persist on this subject, with much talk from each and little listening between," Dr. Blackburn wrote.[20]

In 1980, the president of the National Academy of Sciences, Dr. Philip Handler, criticized the low-fat recommendation making its way into federal nutrition guidelines, testifying before Congress, "What right has the federal government to propose that the American people conduct a vast nutritional experiment, with themselves as subjects, on the strength of so very little evidence?"[21]

But the evidence didn't seem to matter. People went with the scary story about fat — the story they'd been hearing about — and the guy who was telling it.

In 1980, the fat-causes-heart-disease bandwagon got a big boost. The American College of Cardiology was now on board. Soon, the government's dietary recommendations got even stricter on how much fat a person should consume. The WHO adopted the U.S. guidelines. By this time, all public dissent had been quashed. Overnight, farmers who had lived off their livestock were seen as anti-science deviants, rebelling against progress, and threatening public health. Dr. Keys and his wife wrote a cookbook, which became a bestseller. The AHA followed by selling a popular cookbook of its own with the official American Heart Association brand on it. It was the first in a series, beginning in 1973. (As I write this book, I notice that the latest 2024 AHA cookbook library includes another new cookbook bannering "low-cholesterol recipes.") In the U.S., no prominent large medical association dissented from the prevailing view.

The global war on fat seemed to be going great for Dr. Keys and his friends.

But then epidemiologists began to look at obesity and diabetes trends. They noted that after each major low-fat recommendation push, obesity and diabetes in the U.S. accelerated. The first turning point started in 1961 with the first major low-fat recommendation. Rather than reexamine the basis for the recommendation, doctors dug in. When confronted with surging obesity rates, doctors dismissed the possibility that it could be a consequence of eating low-fat food that happened to be loaded with more sugar. To the medical establishment, the reason for the spike was clear: Americans were cheating or noncompliant with doctors' orders. In their paternalistic minds, doctors just needed to push harder.

The First of Three Inconvenient Truths

Soon after Dr. Keys told the world about his hypothesis, he helped launch a study designed to end all studies. It began in the 1960s. Led by his University of Minnesota colleague Dr. Ivan Frantz, the trial enrolled a whopping 9,000 people, randomizing half to a low-fat diet and half to a standard higher-fat diet.[22]

But the results they got were *not* what they were expecting. There were *more* cardiac deaths in the low-fat diet group. More specifically, there were 269 deaths in the low-fat group vs. 248 deaths in people who ate a regular diet, higher in fat.

The results went the wrong way.

It was deeply embarrassing for Dr. Keys, and likely it was for that reason that he removed himself from the study and its results were sequestered. The study, known as the Minnesota Heart Study, would eventually be published 16 years later, in 1989, by Dr. Frantz. Before Dr. Frantz's death, Gary Taubes asked him why he had waited 16 years to publish the results. Frantz replied, "We were just so disappointed in the way they turned out."[23]

That's not how science is supposed to work.

Critics of Dr. Keys would later explain the findings by suggesting low-fat food had higher amounts of refined carbohydrates, known to increase inflammation of the coronary arteries. It's this inflammation that allows for deposition of certain types of lipoproteins, causing plaques and heart attacks.

By the time the Minnesota Heart Study was published in 1989, it was too late. The medical establishment and government health agencies were intoxicated on the thesis that fat was the root of heart disease. Changing the warpath of the medical establishment would be like turning around an aircraft carrier that had been stuck in mud.

Here's one reason why: The year before the Minnesota Heart Study was published, the AHA had announced it would license its "healthy heart" seal to restaurants and food companies for foods that met its guidelines for salt, cholesterol, and fat content.[24] The AHA's president said the program, which was approved by the membership delegates, was a "logical expansion" of its efforts to reduce premature death and disability from heart attack and stroke. In covering the announcement, the *New York Times* parroted the AHA's claim "that dietary control was one of the most effective ways to reduce the risk of cardiovascular disease" and reminded readers that the AHA had been consistent on this recommendation since 1961. It would take Gary Taubes, in his book *Rethinking Diabetes,* and another independent journalist, Nina Teicholz, author of *The Big Fat Surprise,* to expose the dogma, decades later.

The Second Blow

If the Minnesota Heart Study, albeit sequestered, was the first major blow to Dr. Keys, the NIH's Framingham Heart Study, led by researchers at the Harvard School of Public Health, was the second. The largest long-term study ever conducted of heart disease, it began collecting data on diet and health outcomes in 1948. Dr. George Mann, a highly respected Vanderbilt University professor and nutritional biochemist, co-led the study. When he and his team tabulated the results in 1960, it was obvious that saturated-fat intake was *not* causing heart disease. Researchers wrote in an internal document about the potential association between fat intake and heart disease: "No relationship found."[25]

However, this finding was buried in a stack of reports (volume 24 of 26) that was not published in a medical journal; instead, it was made available to some medical school libraries about a decade later. The results did not surface to the public until decades later, in 1992, when a subsequent study director, Dr. William P. Castelli, disclosed them: "The more saturated fat one ate . . . the *lower* the person's serum cholesterol . . . and [they] weighed the *least*."[26] That's 32 years of keeping the public in the dark! The scientific community had been flying blind with no knowledge of either the Minnesota Heart Study nor this Framingham Heart Study.

A lot of bandwagon thinking prevailed in those years.

Dr. George Mann later came out and said he had been forbidden from publishing the early results of the Framingham study back in the 1960s.[27] He was threatened that if he kept up his contrarian behavior, he would never get another grant. And that's exactly what happened. He courageously wrote in 1985 that, "A generation of citizens have grown up since the diet/heart hypothesis was launched as official dogma. They have been misled by the greatest scientific deception in our times: The notion that consumption of animal fat causes heart disease."

Wow. Despite his many accomplishments and high standing as the associate director of the NIH's Framingham Heart Study, medical oligarchs turned on him for the crime of wanting to make the results public. They ruined his career, not inviting him to speak at meetings and conferences, and ending his funding — the lifeline we all need in academic research.

Around this time, new technology came on the scene. Cardiologists began routinely looking at the coronary arteries with catheter technology. They noticed something peculiar: Some patients with high cholesterol would have no blockages and, conversely, some patients with low cholesterol had severe blockages. They began to question conventional wisdom.

The Third Blow

Then the third major blow to the fat hypothesis happened. Remember the NIH's Women's Health Initiative study that was misrepresented to claim that hormone replacement therapy causes breast cancer? Well, four years after that 2002 publication, a separate group of researchers took a look at the same 48,000-woman database to ask a different question: Did women who ate a low-fat diet live longer? The result: They did not.[28]

"A dietary intervention that reduced total fat intake . . . did not significantly reduce the risk of CHD [coronary heart disease] and stroke," the researchers concluded. The study, published in *JAMA,* poured cold water on the fat hypothesis, but, oddly, it was omitted from the summary of scientific evidence compiled by the U.S. government dietary guidelines committee in 2015.

Nina Teicholz pointed out the omission in an article she wrote for the medical journal *BMJ*. She also wrote a *New York Times* op-ed calling out members of the government's 2015 dietary guidelines committee for not disclosing money they had been paid from the food industry. For pointing out those simple facts, she was excoriated by the medical establishment. Scores of scientists signed a petition demanding the *BMJ* retract her article, which the journal refused to do. I was on the *BMJ* editorial advisory committee at the time. I was not involved in the decision but was proud of the bold position the editor in chief took. Too many leaders today cave to this kind of pressure as others put their head in the sand.

Teicholz had not committed research fraud or killed anyone. She had committed a crime far worse: She had embarrassed medical patriarchs.

A distinguished New York University professor of nutrition, Dr. Marion Nestle, condemned Teicholz for her *BMJ* article, telling *Politico,* "What I find so distressing is that this just further confuses the public."[29] I reached out to Dr. Nestle, who is unrelated to the Nestlé corporation but is a giant in the nutrition field, to ask her if Teicholz had said anything that was incorrect. She said no, then quickly pointed out that others were also critical of Teicholz, not just her. Dr. Nestle suggested to me that Teicholz's article had been retracted, but I let her know it had not.

I then asked Dr. Nestle about the 1988

Surgeon General's report that famously recommended a low-fat diet (she had edited the report). When I asked her to point me to the single best study to support the low-fat recommendation, she replied, "I don't think it's one study . . . The studies are hard to do . . . It's what people thought at the time, and it was universally thought at the time." Remarkably, she told me she still believes in the low-fat recommendation. We'll explore the psychology of that mindset in the next chapter. I asked Dr. Nestle to reconcile her view with the above three large studies, none of which found a connection between fat intake and heart disease. Here's how she responded:

"If you think that everybody was wrong . . . then you're looking at an awful lot of people who were delusional, all those people in the American Heart Association, all those people in the National Academy, all those people in the Surgeon General's report. Really? Everybody was crazy? I don't think so."

In other words, everyone believes it so it must be true.

She added that Dr. Keys was a giant, pointing out to me that the government's dietary guidelines "have not changed since 1980 and they're no different from his dietary guidelines in the late 1950s and the reason why they're continuing is because the evidence continues to support them."

I was astonished that she thought the low-fat recommendation still exists in current government dietary guidelines. It doesn't. The 2015 government dietary guidelines committee had actually acknowledged that the low-fat recommendation had moved people to consume foods high in refined carbohydrates, which may have contributed to increased rates of heart disease.

I'm amazed at the legacy of Ancel Keys, despite the scathing critique of his studies and the inability of other studies to confirm his theory. The Minnesota Heart Study, the Framingham Heart Study, and the Women's Health Initiative study were three huge blows, but these revelations came too late. The train had left the station, and there was no stopping it. The AHA was making millions by licensing its low-fat healthy heart seal to food companies and restaurants across America.

Honoring Our High Priests

When Dr. Keys died in 2004, the third most widely read medical journal in the world, the *Lancet,* published a glowing article detailing his many achievements. The tribute did not mention any controversy or that he had used bad science to propagate one of the greatest scientific myths of the modern era.[30] The *New York Times* similarly had a laudatory piece, praising him for "putting saturated fat on the map as a major cause of heart disease."[31]

One of his leading opponents, Dr. Yudkin, who ended up being correct, died in 1995 "a disappointed, largely forgotten man," only recognized 21 years later in the *Guardian* and in books by Gary Taubes.[32] But the work of Dr. Yudkin would be resurrected years after his death by University of California San Francisco pediatric endocrinologist Robert Lustig, who conducted studies validating the refined carbohydrate cause of heart disease. Refined carbohydrates are not the types of sugars found in fruit, which are complex and bound to fiber, resulting in slow absorption in the gastrointestinal tract. Refined carbohydrates instead are sugars and refined grains that have been stripped of all bran, fiber, and nutrients — such as white bread. Over the last 15 years many prominent physicians have come full circle, now recognizing the role of refined carbohydrates, and they have stopped hammering their patients to switch to low-fat foods. Most younger health professionals are in tune with this new science. My cousin Morris, Uncle Sam's son, was one of those doctors.

Dr. Dudley White became known as the father of cardiology in the U.S. He remains a hero at the Massachusetts General Hospital, where annual awards are given in his name and his portrait is prominent in the main gallery. Dr. White did seem to have quietly parted ways with Dr. Keys. In reading his writings later in life, it appears that he felt that he'd been fooled.

Dr. Walter Willett, the most influential nutrition scientist since Dr. Keys, was a staunch enthusiast for Keys's diet. I crossed paths with him at the Harvard School of Public Health, where he was a highly celebrated faculty member (and friendly to students). An epidemiologist, he chaired the nutrition department for 26 years, until 2017. I personally never saw the picture on the wall of his office of him shaking Dr. Keys's hand, but Nina Teicholz told me she has. At the age of 79, he is still on the Harvard faculty.

I remember one lecture he gave when I was a student there. I had no idea what the truth was, so I blindly believed everything he eloquently said. In recent years, people have been highly critical of him receiving millions from the food industry as he downplayed the role of carbohydrates. He literally wrote a textbook of nutrition that was used in schools around the world. Dr. Willett is the #1 most cited researcher in medicine, according to Research.com's list of "Best Medicine Scientists" — generated by calculating an index score of the impact of one's research as measured by how often other science writers cite their research. (Dr. JoAnn Manson of the Women's Health Initiative study on hormone therapy is #5 on that same list.) Looking at the top 100 list, the top five scientists are from Harvard.

Like Dr. Keys, Dr. Willett has had sharp words for people who disagreed with him. He denounced Dr. Katherine Flegal, an epidemiologist at the CDC's National Center for Health Statistics, for publishing a study showing that people who were slightly overweight lived longer.[33] Some have speculated that the finding may be due to people who are slightly overweight having a lower fall risk or more muscle mass.

But Dr. Willett would have none of it. "This study is really a pile of rubbish, and no one should waste their time reading it," he told NPR.[34] He claimed that the media's interest in reporting Dr. Flegal's findings represented a danger to public health, and worried that her study would confuse the public and doctors. In other words, he wanted her canceled. She later wrote in the medical journal that Dr. Willett had led "an aggressive campaign that included insults, errors, misinformation, social media posts, behind-the-scenes gossip and maneuvers, and complaints to her employer."[35] If this charge is true, it suggests that this area of science is not exactly an open forum for the exchange of ideas. It's more a kingdom run by oligarchs.

The story of Dr. Keys and his allies reveals something important about the medical establishment. It shows that a consensus can sometimes be the product of strong internal lobbying by a few highly influential people.

Deep Burn

The AHA propagated the hypothesis of Dr. Keys for 60 years. By picking him over Dr. Yudkin (fat over sugar) they bet on the wrong horse. But more concerning is that rather than making a strong public apology once the data became clear, the organization simply faded back and quietly modified its guidelines many years later.

The AHA's hardline guideline to avoid cholesterol and fat, albeit based on flawed science, has stuck in people's minds. To this day, when overweight people go to their doctor, they are often told to eat low-fat foods. Moreover, most people whose blood tests reveal a high total or LDL cholesterol are told to reduce their cholesterol intake. These recommendations are nothing more than a remnant from a prior era of junk science and groupthink.

The dogma has passed through generations. Given all the conflicting information on food, people tend to believe what their parents taught them. In my case, I was 100% sure that breakfast was the most important meal of the day because that's what my mother told me. I would eat a full breakfast with eggs each morning before school, but later when I fell in love with sugary cereals, I would battle a food coma as I sat in class. I continued to stubbornly believe breakfast is the most important meal of the day even through medical school.

But then a friend showed me where that dogma came from. The concept was invented by the physician Dr. John Harvey Kellogg — the creator of Corn Flakes and other breakfast cereals — as a company marketing campaign.

Cavemen and women didn't wake up to a premade breakfast buffet. They would hunt and gather during the day and eat during the day and at night. Going into a prolonged active digesting mode in the morning after a large breakfast is not ideal. People should be active during the morning to optimize health. These big meals, including massive carbohydrate-loaded school lunches that make children struggle to stay awake in early afternoon classes, are a modern-day invention. Personally, I now eat a small bite and drink for breakfast instead of the large meal that Dr. Kellogg wanted me to eat.

My uncle Sam seemed to be smarter than Dr. Kellogg. Rather than wake up out of bed and stuff himself, he has a quick drink, then goes walking, swimming, and socializing each morning. By late morning, he sits down to enjoy his eggs prepared the way he likes them.

Restoring Objectivity

Just because there is a study to support an idea does not mean the study was designed properly, conducted ethically, or reported accurately. When I hear people making medical claims, I often take a close look at the underlying study used to support them. Sometimes it's strong, or at least intriguing. But other times, the study provides zero support for their claims.

One of my greatest concerns is that today's

public health and medical experts — and certainly the media — have lost the ability to critically appraise research quality. If a shoddy study supports what people already believe, it's hailed as definitive science, but if a strong study conflicts with a foregone conclusion, it's ignored or nitpicked.

What do I mean by nitpick?

When I was a student at the Harvard School of Public Health, we had a standard homework assignment. We would take six studies that had recently been published by *JAMA* and the *New England Journal* and nitpick them to death. We did it as a learning exercise — to examine methods and limitations in studies and reflect on how we would do similar work. We could always do it. *This one didn't provide the height and weight of the patients, this one didn't test the urine of patients to see if they were compliant with their medication,* and on and on. We could always find some way to criticize a study. Our grades depended on it! Of course, many of these studies contained interesting findings. But if we wanted to invalidate the study, we could carpet bomb it with endless minor critiques. In fact, we started with a checklist of 15 elaborate standards and would just go through the list until a study was deficient on one of them. Of course, no study ever published could meet all 15 standards. What I learned was to design research studies optimally, but what was frightening was that I also learned how to destroy any study I didn't like.

This is also how the NIH scores grant proposals to determine which researchers around the country to fund with taxpayer money. If the old belt-and-suspenders professors don't like a new research proposal because it could potentially challenge their own decades-long work, they nitpick it. If it supports their work, they instantly fall in love with it and overlook possible problems with the proposed research.

Medical journals do it, too. I've published extensively in the medical literature, including in all the top medical journals, and been on editorial boards. I'm intimately familiar with scientific standards for publishing research. But in the last few years, I have been shocked to see studies so flawed that the results are rendered invalid, yet they were published in prestigious medical journals and upheld as scientific proof when instead they just support a groupthink narrative. I've also seen sound studies with excellent methods nitpicked when they do not support the popular narrative. Some journals are shameless about it. The medical journal *Nature* openly states on its website that its policy is to remove articles that "might contradict widely accepted public-health advice."

If that policy had been in place during the fat debate, Dr. Yudkin's articles could have been removed for challenging conventional thinking. The same for the researchers that debunked Keys's "Seven Country Study."

The former editor of the *New England Journal,* Dr. Marcia Angell, once told a friend of mine that they were having trouble getting decent articles to publish every week. "Imagine what the other journals are getting!" she said. You'll get to know Dr. Angell better in a few chapters.

As I speak to researchers about these well-known problems, they often tell me how they are afraid to say anything publicly, for fear of being blackballed by the small group of people that control the currency of academic medicine. Every researcher needs the NIH to fund their proposals, and they need medical journals to publish their articles; therefore, medical oligarchs who hold tremendous power are rarely challenged.

To resurrect the scientific method, we need to be objective in how we evaluate research, including research we don't like by people we don't like.

A Great Irony

Almost every day in the hospital, I can see the legacy of Dr. Keys. Whether the medical staff is talking to patients about healthy foods, counseling them to lose weight before surgery, or seeing someone eat a snack or low-fat nutrition bar in the cafeteria, Ancel Keys is everywhere.

A few years ago, I strolled into an open enrollment health benefits fair at my hospital. There were booths with exhibitors explaining each of the health plan offerings, such as dental coverage and retirement benefit options. I gravitated to a booth labeled "Nutrition," where I met two dieticians. I asked them what they were offering, and they kindly explained their nutrition consultation services are available to hospital employees. I then asked what they recommended, theoretically, for an overweight person who was trying to lose weight. They said they would generally recommend that the person eat foods that are low in cholesterol and fat.

Incredible.

I smiled and said thank you. Our hospital has been ranked as number one by *U.S. News and World Report* for 22 years. As my mentor Dr. John Cameron would say when something embarrassing happened at our hospital, "I wonder what's going on at the number-two hospital."

WHAT TO DO?

This chapter is not intended to tell you what to eat. It's to show you how bandwagon thinking can dominate the medical community. Excessive portions of high-fat foods can change your LDL levels on a standard blood test. There may be special situations where a physician may appropriately advise against a high-fat diet and in particular, excessive portions. But on a population level, avoiding dietary cholesterol and saturated fat has *not* been found in several large studies to result in a longer life.

Coronary heart disease is now recognized as a result of general body inflammation which, at the level of the coronary arteries, allows certain types of lipoproteins to deposit. Lipoprotein A (LPa) and Apolipoprotein B (ApoB) are examples of the prime culprits. ApoB is followed more closely in Europe than in the U.S., but every adult in the U.S. should have both checked, in my opinion. You can ask for it the next time your doctor orders a blood test, but make sure they know how to interpret them. ApoB and LPa are probably the best screening tests to evaluate your lipoprotein profile — better than HDL and LDL.

Several studies have found that statins can lower one's mortality. But why? It's been assumed that it's because they lower lipid levels. That may be true, but in reality we don't know if it's due to their lipid-lowering effect or their anti-inflammatory effect. It's likely the latter because statins have been shown to improve survival in people with normal lipoprotein levels.[36] Inflammation is driven by refined carbohydrates, which is why many doctors are now advising patients to limit their intake of refined carbohydrates in their diets as a way to promote heart health.

Statins and other medications can be an effective way for people with a high ApoB level to live longer. For a deeper dive, I recommend the book *Outlive: The Art and Science of Longevity* by Dr. Peter Attia.

In this chapter, we focus on the herd mentality that drives some medical recommendations. The field of medicine certainly needs more doctors with courage like Attia, Yudkin, and Mann to use the scientific method to challenge deeply held assumptions.

A 60-Year Mistake

For about 60 years, the AHA failed to question the dogma that reducing dietary cholesterol and saturated fat lowered heart disease. Today the AHA is starting to come around.

Their website now states, "Fat gets a bad rap even though it is a nutrient we need in our diets."[37] It's like, does a fish know that it's wet?

But many people still promote low-fat, low-cholesterol foods, rather than promoting portion control and whole foods, and limiting refined carbohydrates.

Let's pause for a second and zoom out.

The medical establishment got the primary cause of heart disease wrong for 60 years.

It got hormone replacement therapy wrong for 22 years.

It got antibiotic appropriateness wrong for 60 years.

It got peanut allergy prevention wrong for 15 years.

It got the addictive properties of opioids wrong for 20 years.

This is a partial list of major errors by the medical establishment on leading issues in health. The errors are not oversights of an ancient era; they are avoidable mistakes in modern medicine. The issues could have been resolved with sound research conducted *before* recommendations were made with such absolutism. They are worth describing because the evidence-based corrections of these errors are still not widely known. In the coming chapters, we'll explore the *culture* of medicine that catalyzed groupthink and the paternalism that hammered it in. We'll also ask what we're doing today that could be wrong.

I'm not bitter about these groupthink errors of the medical establishment. My faith teaches me to forgive. The purpose in detailing them is to 1) broaden people's perspective about the range of scientific study on these topics, 2) encourage civil discourse, and 3) encourage an open-minded approach to scientific dialog so that the scientific method can more universally govern our profession.

Ultimately, I'm optimistic about the future of medicine. What is my greatest inspiration for being optimistic? My uncle Sam is back to eating his eggs.

CHAPTER 5

True Believers

Why we resist new ideas

Never underestimate the difficulty of changing false beliefs by facts.

— Henry Rosovsky

For decades, we surgeons have been trained to recognize an inflamed appendix on a CAT scan and then leap into action. Like a swift military operation, I have activated my surgical team hundreds of times to get a patient to the operating room so I could remove their appendix. After doing so many of these procedures, they start to blur together. One night, I found myself at an evening cocktail reception after a long day of doing several emergency appendectomies. While thanking someone for their generosity I absentmindedly added, "If I can ever return the favor, I'd be happy to remove your appendix free of charge."

Then one day, a new study challenged our go-to treatment of this ancient disease.

The study found that a short course of antibiotics alone can cure appendicitis, avoiding the need for surgery. The study seemed to be well conducted, with dramatic results. It felt jarring to be confronted with research that directly went against what I and every other surgeon had been doing for decades.

A few weeks later, I was on call for the emergency room and saw the perfect candidate for the new approach: a young man with early appendicitis.

"My sister's getting married in Boston tomorrow," he told me. "I'd really like to be there."

I was torn. He looked comfortable and barely had any pain. If I operated on him immediately, he'll be laid up in recovery for the next few days and miss his sister's wedding. I decided to tell him about the new study and give him the option: take an antibiotic or have surgery. I explained the risk of antibiotics (including to the microbiome) — but given that it would be a short course of antibiotics that could negate the need for surgery, and that surgery would involve antibiotics anyway, this was one of the appropriate uses I would support.

Because he was not a masochist, he chose no surgery. (Who wouldn't?) So that's what we did. I prescribed him antibiotics, and we waited to see whether or not it worked.

Worried stiff, I checked on him every few hours. At one point, I overheard the emergency department nurses asking, "Why is Dr. Makary incessantly checking in on this one patient who doesn't even look like he needs to be here?"

Within 12 hours, I got a call from his nurse. "He has zero pain and wants to leave." I sent him off to Boston, where, he later told me, he danced up a storm at his sister's wedding. He never needed surgery or got appendicitis again. The new protocol had worked.

The public policy researcher in me stopped to think about the massive implications of this new research for health care: All the cost savings of doing less surgery, how it would help our nursing shortage, and how it could reduce our carbon footprint (hospitals are some of the greatest producers of waste). It could also shorten the daily waitlist of hospitalized patients standing by to have surgery. Approximately 300,000 people come to a hospital with appendicitis each year. It's one of the most common operations in medicine. Broad adoption of this nonoperative approach could have massive implications for health and for health care costs.

I shared my experience with a surgeon

colleague, who is a friend, and asked him what he thought of the new study.

"I don't buy it. I need to see a randomized controlled study," he said.

Several months later, his wish came true. A randomized controlled trial was published in our top surgery journal, showing the same thing: About 75% of people with appendicitis don't need surgery.[1] I emailed him the study and then asked him about it.

"I need to see two randomized controlled trials," he told me.

His response seemed more territorial than objective. The published study was well designed and included one-year follow-up data with excellent results. But then approximately six months later, a second randomized controlled trial came out. It was published in *JAMA* and showed similarly impressive results.[2] I again emailed him the study, then asked him about it in person when I bumped into him.

"I need to see a third randomized controlled trial," he insisted.

What? Now I sensed it was not about the science. I shared with him my experience treating several patients with the new approach, successfully sparing most of them the need for surgery. I also told him that the protocol has long been used in Europe.

But he seemed uninterested. If anything, he seemed annoyed and uncomfortable with what I was saying.

When I asked him what issues he had with the study methodology, it seemed he had not read it. I was curious if his resistance was because he loved being a busy surgeon, or because nearly every surgeon gets paid a bonus based on their number of operations. (I refuse to be on this hamster wheel and do not participate in the annual bonus.) But my colleague had never struck me as the money-hungry type. He was a dependable and honest guy.

Then two years later, a third randomized controlled study was published in another top journal[3] and, separately, *JAMA* published impressive five-year follow-up results of patients who had avoided surgery.[4] Other studies reported the same results in children.[5,6] At this point, it would be unethical to do another similar study and randomize more people to surgery. In a plethora of reproducible studies, the data had spoken. It was no longer an open question.

I went back to my colleague gently and asked him if he had seen all the new studies. I asked him what he thought of them. I named each one, summarizing their results in turn.

"Marty, I just think people are better off with their appendixes out," he replied. Amazing. All the research in the world wouldn't matter. For him, it wasn't a scientific view, it was a belief system. My colleague (now retired) did not want to change his mind.

And he was not alone. Today, about a decade after the first definitive study showing how the non-operative approach works, only about half of surgeons have incorporated it into their practice. The other half still operate on everyone they see with straightforward appendicitis. That means whether or not you go under the knife for appendicitis today in America depends on who's on call when you walk into the emergency department.

Cognitive Dissonance

People are reluctant to change their beliefs. Even highly educated people who are otherwise kind and reasonable can be hostile to new ideas. The psychologist best known for explaining this mystery is the late Dr. Leon Festinger.

Dr. Festinger theorized that people feel discomfort if the beliefs they hold are inconsistent with new information. He postulated that when people are asked to consider a new belief or do something that runs counter to their beliefs, they go into a state of mental conflict. He called the resulting discomfort "cognitive dissonance."

How do people deal with cognitive dissonance? Dr. Festinger observed that they may try to resolve the dissonance by slightly modifying their beliefs to make them fit the new information. Or they resolve the dissonance by denying the new information. He found that people would often convince themselves the new information was actually not different from their preexisting belief at all. Some would twist themselves into a mental pretzel to keep their preexisting belief alive. In short, cognitive dissonance is uncomfortable. Even so, few people are willing to do the hard work of reevaluating their beliefs to account for new information.

In one social experiment, Dr. Festinger and his colleague Dr. James Carlsmith paid people to perform a tedious task for an hour.[7] One group was paid $20 and the other group was paid $1. It turned out that participants who were paid $1 rated the experience as more fun. Why? Because they needed a way to resolve their cognitive dissonance. It's unreasonable to get paid $1 per hour to perform a tedious task. It creates an incongruent situation. So the participants told themselves that it was fun. They might have thought, *It's not so unreasonable to perform a fun task for $1 an hour.*

Dr. Festinger's principle helped me understand why my colleague rejected sound research on a new treatment. Consider, for example, a man who has always believed that his smoking habit is not really that bad for his health. Then he sees new research showing that it *is* bad. He might discredit the study, regardless of its merits, or suggest that it doesn't apply to him because he doesn't smoke exactly the same amount that subjects did in the study. He might even try to argue that he's about to quit so the study of long-term use doesn't apply to him. By reframing things, he can make both thoughts true: Smoking is bad *and* it's not bad for him. According to Dr. Festinger, this type of mental acrobatics is the natural way human beings subconsciously strive to maintain consistency in their views.

Dr. Festinger's theory named an important truth of human psychology. We don't like inconsistent beliefs, so we try hard to resolve them by explaining away the differences.

Effort Justification

The theory was further supported by an experiment by psychologists Drs. Elliot Aronson and Judson Mills.[8] The researchers invited women to participate in a sex discussion group. In order to participate, they first had to pass an initiation test. The women were divided into three groups without even knowing that there were three groups. The first group had a difficult entrance test, the second had an easy test, and the third group had no test. After they were divided, the researchers gave the participants an extremely boring talk about how bees reproduce. The talk was designed to be a disappointment.

The researchers then asked the participants to rate how enjoyable the talk had been. Remarkably, the participants with the harder entrance exam found the talk to be most enjoyable. This became known in psychology as the principle of "effort justification." People who took a hard entrance exam had convinced themselves their hard work served a purpose: It was to earn admission into an enjoyable talk.

Effort justification explains why achieving something in life can cause unnecessary pain. The principle of effort justification to manage cognitive dissonance also explains other excessively difficult rites of passage: fraternity hazing, incessant testing in school, and 36-hour shifts in medical residency. *We* did it in the past, therefore *they* must do it

— precisely to reduce the cognitive dissonance of those in charge.

As a resident who worked 36-hour shifts like generations of doctors before me, I remembered hearing about new research showing that being awake for 36 hours straight resulted in poor motor skills and impaired judgment. The research showed the exhaustion was equivalent to being intoxicated! They wouldn't want us boozing it up in the hospital, but somehow it was okay for all of us to work while exhausted?

Friends asked me why hospitals continued to insist that residents work 36-hour shifts. I had been indoctrinated by a medical culture that said we needed to get abused to make us tough. I actually believed what I was told; the stupor of extreme sleep deprivation was a stress test, like the near-drowning during training of Navy SEALs. It made us stronger. This suggests a bit of a cult mentality, but it is also the only path created by medical high priests to be a surgeon. I watched fellow residents go to the breaking point, engaging in substance abuse, ending relationships, some even committing suicide. Yet we believed somehow that the 120-hour workweek including a couple shifts of 36 hours or more each week was necessary. Senior surgeons who had gone through the rite of passage before us rationalized that sleep deprivation was the only way to follow a patient for their entire hospital stay.

Luckily, some work-hour restrictions were enacted after I finished my residency. Operating "on no sleep" had been considered a badge of honor. It's now rightfully considered reckless. To this day, many who propagated from the 120-hour workweek still insist that those were the "good ol' days" and that today's students and residents need to work harder.

Cognitive dissonance and effort justification explain so much of human behavior. They also explain the perpetuation of medical dogma. These concepts are not just abstract; they affect how we behave today. In my job, we are constantly evaluating new medical interventions, medications, devices, and surgical techniques. Cognitive dissonance is palpable every time we read new studies and discuss them as a medical community. The findings of Dr. Festinger's research are a constant reminder to recognize our natural tendency to discount or alter new information to make it fit what we already believe. We must actively manage and correct that tendency.

It gets really wild when we see just how

far people will take these errant patterns of thinking.

Embedding in a Cult

When Dr. Festinger developed the theory of cognitive dissonance, he had only applied it to past events. He had no way to test it in the real world. But then, sitting at home one day, he read an article in the newspaper about a cult predicting an apocalypse later that year.

The cult members believed that aliens from the planet Clarion were flying over the earth and could see fault lines that would result in a great flood. The messages were relayed through "automatic writing" from the aliens, channeled to the cult's leader, a woman from Chicago who went by Mrs. Martin. She claimed that she had received a message that the catastrophic flood would occur on December 21, 1954, the winter solstice.[9] The good news, she said, was that the aliens communicated that they were coming to rescue her and her followers, picking them up from her house. Cult members, including one physician, prepared for their departure.

Dr. Festinger rushed to embed himself inside the cult to test his hypothesis. He joined psychologists Henry Riecken and Stanley

Schachter in posing as ordinary people with a sincere interest in flying saucers and the cult's beliefs. If his theory was true, once the date had passed, devoted cult members would not admit that their prophecy was false. Instead, they would become more committed.

From inside the cult, he and the other researchers noted that many cult followers had a high degree of belief. They had quit their jobs, dropped out of school, or ended relationships. Most truly believed that a spaceship would pick them up at midnight on that December day.

But when the midnight deadline had passed, devoted cult members were not humiliated, nor did they admit their error. Rather, they dug in. Dr. Festinger had been right. Here's a play-by-play description of the night, adapted from the writings of Dr. Festinger and his colleagues in their book *When Prophecy Fails*:[10]

- December 20. Preparing for the midnight arrival of the spacecraft, cult members remove all metallic items including zippers and bra straps so they would not melt in the spacecraft.
- At midnight, nothing happened. No aliens arrived at the house.

- 12:05 A.M. Still no spaceship. The group sits in the house patiently waiting. One cult member notices that another clock in the room reads 11:55. The clock had been set ten minutes behind, but the group agrees that it is not yet midnight.[11]
- 12:10 A.M. The second clock now shows that it's midnight. Still no alien delegation to pick them up. The flood that was to destroy the earth is supposed to happen by morning.
- 12:30 A.M. Someone bangs on the door. The group thinks it could be the alien pick up. It turns out to be some children.
- 4:00 A.M. The group has been sitting in anticipation. The group stays in place in bewilderment. Then Mrs. Martin, the cult leader, begins to cry.
- 4:45 A.M. A message by "automatic writing" is sent directly to Mrs. Martin. It says that the God of Earth has decided to spare the planet from destruction. The reason according to Mrs Martin: "it was this little group spreading light here that prevented the flood."
- Later that afternoon. The media calls. The group engages with them and

> begins a publicity campaign to spread its message to the world.

The conversations that Dr. Festinger and his colleagues recorded tell us more about human reasoning than any MRI could. The cult members that had the strongest beliefs before the apocalypse date became stronger in their conviction. They also increased their recruiting efforts to attract people to join the cult.

Some lukewarm believers abandoned the cult that night, but the researchers observed something interesting. The physician member described how he was in too deep to not keep going. After the prophecy did not come true, the physician said that night, "I've turned my back on the world, I can't afford to doubt, I have to believe . . . I've taken an awful beating in the last few months . . . I can't afford to doubt." Dr. Festinger had predicted that devoted believers would amp up their beliefs after the prophecy was proven wrong. And that's exactly what happened.

In this book, we examine how new information is received in medicine. Dr. Festinger would not be surprised to see the modern-day medical establishment clinging to their deeply entrenched dogmas. As I've shared the topics in this book with colleagues, I've seen Festinger's principles at work. I'm not saying my medical colleagues are like brainwashed cult members scanning the skies for aliens. But the same psychological tendencies seem to apply universally.

For example, when I told a doctor friend that there is no good evidence that HRT causes breast cancer, he responded by saying, "How can that be if breast cancer has hormone receptors on it?" After I explained the studies to him, he continued to find reasons to object: "Why take the risk since there are no benefits to HRT, right?" I could see the gears in his brain trying to resolve the conflict. I then explained how many studies showed that HRT prevents heart attacks, bone fractures, and cognitive decline. After the conversation, he said there might be rare instances when HRT might make sense. This was textbook cognitive dissonance, an intellectual feast for Festinger had he been alive to watch. Similarly, many smart people have had trouble accepting the new science on how antibiotics may harm the microbiome and contribute to chronic disease. "It's because of junk food," one doctor told me. After I showed him the big study on the topic, he said, "Okay, it's junk food and the microbiome." He may be right, but observing his cognitive dissonance was astounding.

In the case of the peanut allergy saga, cognitive dissonance explains why Dr. Gideon Lack was accused of being anti-breast-feeding simply for suggesting the early introduction of peanut products, eggs, and milk at 3 to 6 months of age. He was the furthest thing from it, being a staunch advocate of breast-feeding. He did not believe both were mutually exclusive, as some assumed.

Cognitive dissonance also explains why people rejected the scientists who challenged Dr. Ancel Keys, and why people tend to be fixated on certain diets despite having little knowledge about how they work. In the next few chapters, you will see even more striking cognitive dissonance play out in major national health debates. This book does not discuss the Covid pandemic (people have become too tribal on the topic), but you may have seen cognitive dissonance rear its head on that subject as well.

Festinger's theory is a reminder to us all. We need to constantly maintain a willingness to be open-minded, even if we are deeply invested in a particular belief or position. Doing so requires active effort.

Whether we might be evaluating new information at work, learning something new in everyday life, or pursuing scientific truth, we should remember that progress comes not from the comfort of fitting new ideas into our existing beliefs, but from being uncomfortable by holding our beliefs loosely enough that they can be aligned with new information, when necessary.

How to Be Less Biased

I can be guilty of bias myself. My research colleagues like to poke fun at me for it. We'll be brainstorming ideas for new research and sometimes, I'm told, I can be quick to shoot them down. One of my colleagues will share an idea and I might say, "That's not interesting, we're not doing that." My colleagues say I often use that phrase. While I don't remember saying it that often, other phrases they report coming out of my mouth are "Then we might as well measure the average size of stones on the street" or "I'd rather study how many die each year from a coconut falling on their head." They're right. I like to think my research students and fellows appreciate the directness, but it can come off as hubris. My co-leader, Dr. Caitlin Hicks, and I might hear dozens of new pitches in our weekly meeting, which always has a full agenda. I could be kinder in pointing out the limitations of each idea that we don't want to pursue. The feedback reminded me that we all have preconceived biases, and for me, it has come out in our research ideas meeting.

People who actively work to be open and objective are impressive. They are also easy to spot. They surprise people with their positions on different issues. They don't hop on bandwagons without compelling evidence. And they possess the courage to challenge assumptions and swim against the current. Attorney (and later president) John Adams, for instance, was a supporter of the American Revolution, yet he defended British soldiers in court for acting in self-defense at the Boston Massacre in 1770. Such people are committed to honesty and objectivity, even when it requires straddling opposing ideological camps.

One mentor of mine, who has often demonstrated an impressive level of impartiality, is Dr. John Cameron, our former department chair. It wasn't just in his clinical decision making. When he would hear that a professional athlete was rumored to be in trouble with the law, for example, he would always say, "Let's not make a judgment without having all the facts." That's impressive.

Resisting our natural tendency to reject or reframe information to make it fit our preexisting ideas is important. It also makes for good character. We should all recognize these implicit tendencies and actively work to remain objective. In fact, it's a hallmark trait of many innovators and great leaders. In science, it enables the discovery of truth.

CHAPTER 6

Bad Blood

How the medical establishment actually works

A person with a new idea is a crank until the new idea succeeds.

— Mark Twain

As a fresh med school grad, Don Rucker walked into clinic determined to do good. The packaging folds on his white coat and the pens overflowing his pocket were a dead giveaway that he was a newly minted doctor. Dr. Rucker, who was working at the University of California San Diego, was a bright-eyed, athletic young man. Like most new doctors, he wanted to make a difference.

This wasn't just any clinic in any city. It was the "gay diseases" clinic (yes, believe it or not that's what the doctors called it) in San Diego — a city with a sizable gay community.

The year was 1981, and an epidemic was rapidly unfolding. That summer, 139 gay men had been reported[1] to be immunocompromised with a rare type of infection called pneumocystis, a form of pneumonia. Other gay men had "crypto." No, they were not currency traders; they had an infection called cryptosporidium, a microscopic parasite that causes watery diarrhea and a persistent cough. These infections were opportunistic, occurring in those with an acutely compromised immune system — a constellation of findings that would soon be called AIDS. Public outcry called for rapid research to understand why it was spreading so fast.

One day while out for a run in San Diego's Balboa Park after a full day at the hospital, Dr. Rucker noticed a long line of people waiting outdoors to donate blood at the blood center across the street. As he ran closer, he recognized some of them. They were his patients: IV drug users and gay men he had just seen in clinic or the emergency department. Some had the novel constellation of symptoms. He also knew some had endocarditis (an infection of the heart valve), hepatitis, or anal warts.

Dr. Rucker recounted the scene to me while we met at a diner in Arlington, Virginia: "'Oh no,' I said to myself. 'Whatever is causing this disease is almost certainly in their blood, and now would likely spread to others.'" He added, "Unless you have zero understanding of basic biology, it was very obvious."

Dr. Rucker was no infectious diseases expert, but he had common sense. When examining these patients in clinic, Dr. Rucker would sometimes notice open anal wounds associated with gay sex, suggesting a mode of transmission of the novel outbreak. Another giant clue was the observation that IV drug users who shared needles (and were not gay) were also contracting the disease. Using these few data points, Dr. Rucker deduced that the cause of this deadly disease — soon to be recognized as HIV — was bloodborne.

Dr. Rucker learned another shocking fact about his infected clinic patients that were donating blood. They were not *volunteering* to donate blood — they were being paid to.

"Marty, at that time, the Red Cross paid people to donate blood, specifically plasma, so many poor people would routinely do it, including IV drug users who did it to make money to eat, and for some, to support their drug habit," Dr. Rucker told me. Some of Dr. Rucker's HIV patients were pumping the virus into the blood supply every few months once their blood volume returned to normal.

Like a metronome, his clinic patients

showed up to donate regularly, getting paid each time. In fact, Dr. Rucker quickly learned that for some of them, donating blood was their only job.

Dr. Rucker's instincts were correct: HIV was rapidly spreading through donated blood. But the medical establishment denied the problem, repeatedly downplayed the risks, and refused to effectively screen blood donors. It would be *seven more years* before the U.S. FDA would require America's blood banks to test donated blood, even though Stanford scientists had developed a basic test to screen blood just months after Dr. Rucker's 1981 Eureka moment.

Prominent doctors nationwide agreed with Dr. Rucker's belief that the cause of AIDS was bloodborne. At a July 27, 1982, meeting of the U.S. Public Health Service for blood bankers, some doctors at the meeting sounded the alarm that hemophilia patients, who are often transfused, were getting infected with AIDS after receiving infected blood.

Many other forums had doctors also literally crying bloody murder about the lack of screening based on health and risk factors. Tragically, those voices were ignored. For the vast majority of blood banks in America, nothing changed: No common-sense policies were instituted beyond a few generic precautions implemented very slowly and sporadically.

From the time of Dr. Rucker's realization, it would take nine years until detailed questioning of blood donors to screen for their risk factors would be instituted at all U.S. blood donation sites. In the interim, the public was repeatedly reassured not to worry. Getting a blood donation was said to be "safe."

A Moral Dilemma

One day in the hospital, Dr. Rucker faced a dilemma. He encountered a patient who had experienced a gastrointestinal bleed and had a low level of red blood cells. Giving the patient two units of blood without presenting any alternative option was standard protocol at the time.

But Dr. Rucker knew the blood supply was probably infected with some pathogen that was causing AIDS, so he didn't want to do it. Instead Dr. Rucker gave the patient iron tablets, a common alternative to giving blood, and told him to give him a call if he got worse. Feeling fine and anxious to leave the hospital, the patient was grateful.

The next morning on rounds, Dr. Rucker presented the case to his senior attending physicians. They yelled at him. Any patient with similarly low blood levels must be transfused, they said. Dr. Rucker explained his concerns about the infectious risks to the blood supply, but his seniors would have none of it. They cut him off and scolded him, demanding that he immediately order a STAT blood transfusion of two units for his patient, even though the patient had no complaints. When Dr. Rucker went back to tell his patient what he'd been ordered to do, the room was empty. The patient had left the hospital against medical advice. He never needed the transfusion.

As Dr. Rucker shared his story with me, we laughed about how it always had to be "two units" of blood. The medical culture insisted on it! Nearly every doctor, including myself, had been taught this illogical dogma. Doctors who transfused a single unit were seen as "weak." In addition to this dogma, we were all taught — incorrectly — to transfuse all patients with a hematocrit (red blood cell level) test below 30%. Turns out that the sacred number 30% came from two doctors: Drs. Adams and Lundy had proposed "the 30 rule" back in 1942.[2] It stuck. And became more legendary than Bigfoot. (Everyone believed in it, even though no one had evidence to support it.)

The 30% threshold ended up being the unquestioned blood transfusion trigger for the good part of a century, even appearing in consensus transfusion guidelines as recently as 2012.[3,4] It was pounded into me during my residency. Once I witnessed a senior attending physician mock a resident for not transfusing a stable patient with a hematocrit of 29, just below the magic 30 number. He branded the resident as a sly assassin, calling him "Double-O-Seven."

It's amazing. Many patients receiving HIV-laden blood never even needed the transfusion. And when doctors gave patients two units (just to honor the two-unit-tradition) when they only needed one, we effectively doubled their risk of getting HIV. One meta-analysis of studies published between 1995 and 2005 found that up to 40% of transfusions in the U.S. were unnecessary.[5] When I've heard public service announcements of a "critical blood shortage in your area" I've often thought it might be more accurate to say there's a "critical blood overuse crisis in your area."

Within months after Dr. Rucker's principled refusal to order blood to a stable patient who didn't need it, doctors nationwide were reading CDC reports of patients who had contracted AIDS from a blood transfusion. The most harrowing case was a 20-month-old baby. But remarkably, for most of that decade after Dr. Rucker spoke up about the safety of the blood supply in 1981, he witnessed medical leader after medical leader reassuring the public not to worry about getting AIDS from a blood transfusion.

The Chorus

For much of that decade, America's medical establishment closed ranks and insisted that getting HIV from blood transfusions was either impossible or extremely rare.

A group of doctors from around the country recommended restricting blood donations from high-risk people at a panel discussion hosted by the CDC in January 1983. But the medical establishment dismissed the idea. In a joint statement, the American Red Cross, the American Association of Blood Banks, and the Council of Community Blood Centers rejected the doctors' proposal. They insisted it was "still unproven," "inconclusive," and that "there is no absolute evidence that AIDS is transmitted by blood or blood products."

Sure, maybe it wasn't "absolute," but there were documented cases of AIDS being contracted after a blood transfusion in people with no other exposures to the virus. A lot of lives would have been saved if the medical establishment had just used a little common sense.

The organizations insisted that "direct or indirect questions about a donor's sexual preference are inappropriate."[6]

Later that year the same three blood groups published another joint statement, conceding that while it was possible to get AIDS from a blood transfusion, the risk was miniscule. "The facts do not justify these concerns," the statement said. "Data accumulated over the last three years indicate that the possible occurrence of AIDS in transfusion recipients is on the order of one case per million patients transfused."[7]

Also in 1983, the NIH's deputy clinical director of intramural research for the National Institute of Allergy and Infectious Diseases (NIAID), Dr. Anthony Fauci, weighed in. He issued a statement, with other government officials cosigning, stating that "AIDS is transmitted sexually; less frequently through blood or blood products," and concluding that "the risk of acquiring AIDS through a blood transfusion is extremely small."[8]

At an August 1983 Congressional hearing, Dr. Joseph Bove, Yale professor and director of the Yale–New Haven Hospital blood bank, also used the "one in a million" estimate in his testimony. "If AIDS can be spread by transfusion, what we know now suggests that the risk is minimal," he said. "The incidence will be less than one in a million."

To underscore his point, Dr. Bove included a table with his testimony to compare the risk of a blood transfusion to other "acceptable" risks of dying due to rare events.[9] The table showed:

Transfusion transmitted AIDS	1:1,000,000 (perhaps)
Appendectomy death rate	1:5,000
Automobile racing deaths per person per year	1:10,000
Earthquake deaths per person per year (California)	1:588,000

See how silly it is to be concerned about getting AIDS from a blood transfusion, the table seemed to say. You'd be more likely to die from an earthquake!

To help calm the uproar of concern, New York's top public health official, Dr. David Axelrod, said in a June 21, 1983, statement, "We believe blood transfusions do not present a risk."

Dr. Axelrod was New York's commissioner of health and the AIDS Task Force chairman for the State of New York. "There is no credible evidence," he said, "that what we commonly call AIDS is actually a communicable disease. Yet it is frequently being defined as an infectious or communicable disease, resulting in escalating fears about AIDS spreading . . . through blood transfusions."[10]

The commissioner declared that "ignorance, fear, and misinformation are threatening to overtake science," insisting that "AIDS can only be transmitted through homosexual activity and IV drug use . . . Other risks are not significant."

Advocacy groups for people with hemophilia were voicing the greatest concern about the safety of blood transfusions. Hemophilia is a bleeding disorder, so patients with severe cases often need frequent transfusions to manage their disease. People with severe hemophilia might need a transfusion every few months, and thus they were viewed as canaries in the coal mine in terms of assessing the risk of contracting HIV from the blood supply. Dr. Axelrod pointed to only 14 of the nation's roughly 15,000 people with hemophilia who had contracted AIDS. Not only was his estimate way off, but, remarkably, he seemed to blame the patients with hemophilia themselves for having AIDS. They "may be characterized as a group whose immune system is compromised by an inherent defect," he postulated.[11] Amazing that New York's top health official would say this one year after the CDC reported the death of a San Francisco infant after transfusion from a donor who later died of AIDS. An objective, scientific mind (unaffected by medical field politics) would have likely concluded that such a direct association was causal until proven otherwise.

As late as June 1983, many medical organizations were putting out statements downplaying the risk of getting AIDS from a blood transfusion. That month, the New York State Council on Human Blood and Transfusion Services *unanimously* passed a resolution stating that: "Analysis of all the data collected to date has demonstrated no significant risk for recipients of blood or blood products for contracting the acquired immune deficiency syndrome (AIDS)."

Around the same time, the American Red Cross discouraged "directed donations" — people donating blood for a specific loved one so that the patient doesn't have to receive blood from the general donor pool. However, at the time, directed donations would have been a good idea since the medical establishment was not being straightforward about the risks.

"There is no evidence to support that these 'directed donations' are safer than those available through the community blood bank," the American Red Cross said in a statement.

A year later, Dr. Fauci gave a speech at the NIH acknowledging that contracting AIDS through a blood transfusion was possible but rare. He said the risk was lower than that of dying from getting the wrong blood type due to a clerical error. "The chances of getting AIDS from a transfusion are less than the chances of somebody mixing up the blood and giving you the wrong blood and you're winding up with a transfusion reaction and dying from it. So, the fact is, from an epidemiological standpoint we must be aware of that, but the risk is not great. So the fear of getting a blood transfusion is unwarranted."[12]

The media parroted whatever health authorities said, rarely challenging them or publishing quotes from dissenting experts. *Time* magazine reported in April 1985 that only 142 Americans had contracted AIDS from a blood transfusion, representing a tiny fraction of the 9,600 people who had AIDS in the U.S.[13] In other words, it was such a small percentage that people didn't need to worry about it.

But that same year, an HIV test became available. The more Americans got tested, the more those estimates proved to be tragically wrong. Sixty-three percent of people with hemophilia had become infected with HIV. Essentially all died quickly.[14] In addition, another 4,619 people who did not have hemophilia got the virus from blood transfusions. Another report put the number at 29,000.[15] Both of these estimates are thought to be a massive undercount. Many transfusion recipients were never tested because they were poor, had limited access to care, suffered from addictions, or were noncompliant with care recommendations. Approximately half of those who contracted HIV from a transfusion died within six months, suggesting even more died before they were diagnosed.

Two years prior, in 1983, the American Red Cross told the public that the risk of contracting AIDS from a blood transfusion was "one in a million."[16] The widespread access to testing revealed the true risk at the time was 380 times higher.

Nearly an entire generation of people with severe hemophilia died — a second epidemic.

One *Los Angeles Times* writer referred to it as the "hemophilia holocaust."[17]

The devastation to the hemophilia population was so vast that the disease appeared to be less common for a while. Dr. Rucker recalls how by the late 1980s and into the 1990s, he rarely saw people with the condition. The medical profession had nearly exterminated a generation of people with severe hemophilia.

Medical Paternalism

Why did the medical establishment refuse to effectively screen the blood supply for years after Dr. Rucker's initial observations?

Because it had already made up its mind. Anyone opposing the dogma was excluded. It would be easy to conclude that these medical authorities were arrogant, which may be true. But they also had a good motive: to show support for the life-saving invention of blood donation.

They worried that if they did not provide unified support, people within the general population might choose *not* to get a blood transfusion and could die. Any controversy might also scare off people from donating. Put simply, blood donation and transfusions relied on broad public participation. Anything that dared to question its benefit was regarded as a threat to the institution of blood banking. Their highest priority was to maintain full confidence in the blood bank, which meant assuring the public that no one should worry about contracting HIV.

TODAY

This groupthink reflected a paternalism that plagues modern medicine. It's the same paternalism that opposed allowing women to do their own pregnancy testing until 1976. Women can't handle this information on their own, doctors argued. We must have documentation of their test result in the medical record, they said. Allowing them to get results without a doctor was unacceptable.

Similarly, once an HIV test was developed, the medical establishment blocked attempts for people to test themselves or even get their results on their own. Between 1985 and 2012, Americans were not allowed to get the results of an HIV test without a doctor telling them the results. A few months into the Covid pandemic, Dr. Shantanu Nundy and I proposed in a *Washington Post* article that people be able to test themselves with an at-home test. Some in the medical establishment responded by saying that most people were incapable of reliably testing themselves, and they also may not know what to do with the information they got, thus, people should only be tested at designated centers.

This battle for patient rights plays out every day in America. Even today, patients evaluated for an organ transplant are not able to see where they stand on the waitlist. Sometimes, people are not even on the list and don't know. If you're on the standby list for an upgrade on an airplane, you see where you are, but if you're waiting for an organ, the medical transplant community has no such list where you can see your position.

Medical paternalism still looms large. In recent years, the American Medical Association has been lobbying against patients having full access to all their test results in real time, despite this being a right granted every American in the 21st Century Cures Act enacted by Congress in 2016. On September 30, 2020, California signed into law a provision blocking real-time patient access to test results until a doctor reviews the results first. Specifically, the new law states that test results "shall be reported to the patient within a reasonable time period after the test results are received by the health care professional."[18] California's physician trade association, the California Medical

Association, sponsored the bill and boasted on their website that the new law is "allowing physicians time to interpret potentially life-changing test results before releasing them to the patient electronically."[19] So the next time you learn that your test results are back but that you can't see them yet, you can thank the medical establishment's powerful lobbyists.

I get the motivation behind such bills. We doctors don't want to be bothered with patient calls about tests we haven't looked at yet. But blocking patients' access to their own health information is not the answer.

A Patriot Emerges

In October 1983, almost two years after Dr. Rucker and other doctors could see that the blood supply was not safe, an American hero emerged. Dr. Ed Engleman, a highly driven, 29-year-old doctor at Stanford Medical Center's blood bank, made a lifesaving discovery. He realized that people with AIDS had an abnormal ratio of one white blood cell type relative to another. (The normal ratio of T-helper cells to T-suppressor cells was reversed in AIDS patients.) He and his colleagues quickly developed a screening test for the disease. It cost only about $10 and took about 15 minutes to get the results, and based on their experience at Stanford it was effective. Excited about the implications for society, Dr. Engleman diligently prepared a presentation for the laboratory medicine doctors at the University of California San Francisco.

But as Dr. Engleman explained his new test to screen blood, the audience of several hundred scientists and blood bank officials turned hostile. They did not like what he was proposing. A test for the novel AIDS disease was an acknowledgement that there was a risk. It could alarm the public, they thought. So they tore him to pieces.

"I gave this talk, thinking that it would be cheered," Dr. Engleman later said. "But the opposite happened: They were horrified and felt this was the worst thing ever."

A Stanford pathology resident and postdoc in Dr. Engleman's lab described the event as walking into a firing squad.

"Ninety-eight percent of people involved in the blood-banking world circled the wagons and argued that there was no proof the disease was spread by transfusions and that screening would create a blood shortage," he told Stanford historian Ruthann Richter. "They didn't like the idea of blood banks being associated with this horrible, scary, deadly illness."[20]

Dr. Engleman submitted an abstract on the Stanford test for presentation at the conference for the American Association of Blood Banks. Though abstracts are routinely accepted for the meeting, his did not make the cut. The industry didn't want to acknowledge the problem.

I'm not surprised. In my experience, some conferences accept abstracts based on who the senior author is. Even today, at conferences like the prestigious Southern Surgical Association, you can't even have an abstract considered for the conference program unless one of the authors has passed an arduous application process to become a member first.

A formal HIV test would be developed the following year, but effective screening for HIV in donated blood did not occur for years after Dr. Engleman's discovery. Tens of thousands of Americans contracted HIV from blood transfusions, but at Stanford, Dr. Engleman and his colleagues had implemented their screening test. Stanford became the first U.S. blood bank to screen for HIV, testing blood on approximately 20,000 donors each year.

The result: Stanford prevented many patients from getting HIV.

Beware the Phrase "There is no evidence"

At the same time Stanford doctors were trying to get blood banks to adopt a $10 test to screen for HIV, medical leaders were still insisting, "There is no evidence that HIV can be spread through a blood transfusion." As a result, this flawed guidance was repeated by many doctors when patients asked them about the risk.

Saying "there is no evidence" to silence contrary opinions is an old game. The phrase can be misleading. It is often assumed that "no evidence" means medical professionals have found *evidence that there's no correlation*. I've seen this conflation thousands of times in the hospital. Doctors sometimes use the phrase "There is no evidence to support . . ." to dismiss any idea they don't like or understand, like the role of food or vitamins in health.

When it comes to scientific correlations, the absence of evidence is not evidence of absence. Having no research findings on a topic doesn't mean it's not true. It means it's unknown. Patients can get hoodwinked. I've even seen the phrase weaponized in medical debates to dismiss new ideas. A lack of evidence could simply be a result of there being no research funding allocated to study the matter.

The absence of evidence is often related to the gatekeeping of medical journals, whose perverse incentives may undermine the public good. The *New England Journal* refused to publish the first report of a case of AIDS from a blood transfusion.[21] Some have suggested they did so because the case had already been reported to the CDC and the *New England* likes to always be first.

Sometimes the journals can even suppress scientific discoveries when they should be reporting them. The *New York Times* reported that early in the AIDS epidemic university scientists who had "uncovered clues pointing to a potentially new AIDS-like virus . . . had not shared that information with health officials because they were holding it for publication in scientific journals."[22]

I'm not surprised by this type of behavior. Having personally published over 250 peer-reviewed articles in medical journals, I've been routinely threatened by medical journal editors that if I released any of the findings to the public before the journal's publication date (often several months after submission), I'd be subject to the professional equivalent of the electric chair. They'd probably say this even if my article had a cure for cancer. A similar penalty is often applied if you fail to use the correct font or margins or slightly exceed the word limit (even though journals are now posted online with unlimited space).

So if you've discovered a medical breakthrough that helps patients, you must wait until your annual medical conference or the several months it takes a medical journal to publish it, a ritual that has paralyzed active policy debates on Capitol Hill.

Too often a small group of like-minded editors makes the rules and tightly controls what information gets presented to doctors and the public. The *New England Journal,* for example, has been controlled by a non-diverse group for most of my career. For most of its history, the editorial board had zero diversity. Then in the year 2020, out of 51 editors, one was African American and one was Hispanic, according to an analysis by Dr. Raymond Givens published on the Stat website.[23]

Getting a study published in *JAMA* or the *New England Journal* is rocket fuel for your academic career. One *JAMA* or *New England Journal* study might earn you tenure, a meteoric rise to a department chair position, or a dean job. Most academic physicians will go their entire career without ever publishing once in either of these top journals. In my time at Harvard and Johns Hopkins, I've seen doctors hang a beautifully matted and framed copy of their *JAMA* or *New England Journal* article in their office. Academics consider it a badge of honor.

But editorial board appointments are often based on cronyism, which is why so many *New England Journal* editors are friends and former classmates or colleagues at Harvard or its affiliate hospitals. I saw this firsthand as a student at Harvard, where the *New England Journal* offices are on the second floor of the Harvard Medical School library.

Being a journal editor is a powerful post. Even though it's a part-time job, most editors never step down, and instead serve indefinite terms with their friends. It's okay for a homogenous group of doctors to have their own private medical journal board, but readers should know that their research selections are influenced by a self-affirming bubble effect.

ARTHUR ASHE

Arthur Ashe would have had his life saved by Dr. Rucker's cautious approach to blood transfusion. Ashe, one of the greatest tennis players and civil rights leaders of his day, underwent a major heart operation in 1983, nearly three years after Dr. Rucker and others knew the blood supply was not safe.

Following the surgery, doctors gave the 39-year-old tennis icon HIV by giving him a blood transfusion. Ashe, who had been instrumental in ending apartheid in South Africa by calling to ban the country from international sports competition, survived two heart operations and the civil rights era, but succumbed to HIV in 1993. His official cause of death might have read pneumonia, but in reality it was a preventable medical mistake. To this day, the U.S. Open main stadium in Flushing, New York is named after the tennis great.

Scientific ignorance about the blood supply spreading HIV went on for years. Routine operations that used blood from donors were now far more dangerous than the mortality risk being quoted to the patient during the informed-consent process. People were dying not from the disease that had brought them to care, but from the care itself.

The World Followed

The American medical establishment has a lot of clout worldwide. When other countries struggle with questions of what to do, they often look to the U.S.

While the U.S. finally changed their practice to test donated blood for HIV, other countries were slower to implement the change, after the initial assurances.

As late as 2007, a report on the safety of blood banks in China by the independent group *Asia Catalyst* found that "today, China's blood supply remains dangerously unsafe. Around the country, patients who check into hospitals for routine surgery may check out with HIV/AIDS as a result of hospital blood transfusions"[24]

China also had another problem emblematic of what many poor countries experience. Some doctors reuse needles, and medical suppliers often rinse and resell them without disinfecting. It is estimated that more than half of the Chinese population became infected with hepatitis for this reason.[25]

Celebrating Too Early

Widespread blood testing for the evidence of HIV — using a test that detected HIV antibodies — began in July 1985. And two and a half years later (by January 5, 1988) the FDA required all blood banks to test for anti-HIV antibodies.[26]

The risk of getting AIDS from a transfusion was a thing of the past, according to the message trumpeted by the medical establishment and media. The blood supply was perfectly safe, as the medical establishment declared. But it wasn't. It was simply less dangerous. The testing in place missed as many as 1 in 25 units of blood with HIV.[27] Keep in mind that doctors routinely transfused blood in multiples of two units because dogma held that giving one unit was weak. (I once transfused a young trauma patient 48 units.)

In addition, the HIV test had a blind spot. It takes the body several weeks to generate antibodies. As a result, bags of HIV-laden donated blood flew under the radar of testing. One report found that approximately 500 Americans got HIV from blood in the years *after* universal blood bank testing.

Dr. Ross Eckert, a professor at Claremont McKenna College who served on the FDA's Blood Product Advisory Committee, was a vocal critic of the medical establishment's tardy and arrogant response to screening the blood supply for AIDS. "The evidence shows that the experts managed risk poorly and spread AIDS unnecessarily," he said. He pointed out in many publications that infectious risks in transfused blood lingered for years. Dr. Eckert wrote that *after* a screening test began to be implemented, it did not eliminate the risk. Instead, he wrote, it "reduced the risk markedly to perhaps 1 in 7,100 patients during 1985 to 1989."[28]

Given that about half of all ICU patients got a blood transfusion and many received several, that risk added up.[29]

In my world, that risk is high. When I counsel patients before surgery, I routinely tell them about a roughly 1 in 100,000 risk of dying from general anesthesia. Some patients ask me more about that risk, and we have a conversation weighing those risks against the potential benefits of the operation. That's proper informed consent. But many people given blood transfusions were never made aware of the risks. They would look up at their IV pole and see blood dripping in. It was not until the year 2000 that blood transfusions required a signed consent form.[30]

Individual blood donors were never asked directly about their sexual preference or promiscuity from 1983 to 1990, Dr. Eckert said. The FDA recommended "voluntary self-exclusion" by donors in March 1983, but that just included a pamphlet handed to donors and a consent form. High-risk people donated even though they were given the pamphlet, he added. In 1988, the U.S. Public Health Service found "recognized deficiencies" in the system to educate donors about risk behaviors. A CDC study in 1988–89 showed that almost two thirds donated even though they knew they had engaged in high-risk conduct, Dr. Eckert wrote in a law review article on the subject.[31]

Blood transfusions save lives. I've seen it. But we also now know of other small risks. They can weaken one's immune system and have a potential risk of passing prion proteins, which are not screened for but which caused an outbreak of Creutzfeldt-Jakob disease in the UK.[32] The honest way to talk to patients about a transfusion is to weigh the potential necessity, discuss safe alternatives, and explain that the known risks are small.

Admitting "we don't know" takes humility, but isn't that an essential trait of great doctors? It takes humility to be honest with your patients. It takes humility to know when to get help from another doctor. And it takes humility to accept that the medical dogma pounded into you just might be wrong. But how does one learn humility in a classroom?

Silver Lining

For most of the first decade of the HIV epidemic, Dr. Rucker and other doctors on the front lines of medicine witnessed the remarkable arrogance of a medical establishment ignoring data and plowing over dissent. My dad was a hematologist at the time, treating hemophilia patients in Pennsylvania. He echoed Dr. Rucker's observation: "Always consider risks that are known and risks that are unknown," he said while talking to me about the HIV outbreak.

One of the casualties of the HIV- and hepatitis-contaminated blood in the 1980s was a child named Eric Winer. Born with hemophilia, he contracted both HIV and hepatitis C from a blood transfusion.[33] When he tested positive he did not tell a lot of people, given the intense social stigma of being HIV-positive. Eric had both good doctors and bad doctors take care of him. He was struck by how some of his doctors were great listeners while others couldn't wait to get out of the room. Eventually he went to medical school and became a hematologist–oncologist. Inspired by his own journey, he went on to be an outspoken advocate for listening to what patients want instead of simply telling them what they need to do. He also became a champion for sticking to the principles of science, and for lifting the stigmas doctors can place on patients, even unintentionally.

Dr. Winer became a highly accomplished physician-scientist at the Dana-Farber Cancer Institute in Boston and now leads the Yale Cancer Center. He has influenced tens of thousands of medical students and professionals. In 2020, he received the William Silen Lifetime Achievement in Mentoring Award from Harvard Medical School. In 2023, demonstrating tremendous humility, he shared his powerful personal testimony as a patient in his presidential address as the newly inducted president of the American Society of Clinical Oncology, the world's largest oncology medical association. He continues to be a force for good in changing the culture of medicine.

As for Dr. Rucker, his good instincts would take him far in life. In addition to being an emergency medicine physician, he went on to study medical informatics. As the director of the Office of the National Coordinator for Health Information Technology at the U.S. Department of Health and Human Services, he led national efforts to allow patients to get their electronic medical records digitally *without* requiring them to ask permission.

CHAPTER 7

A Warm Welcome

Rethinking how we bring babies into the world

The true measure of any society can be found in how it treats its most vulnerable members.

— Mahatma Gandhi

I didn't sleep a wink the night before.

Like most medical students on their first day of their obstetrics rotation, I had been consumed with one thought: *Babies are slippery, I hope I don't drop one!* Being a student felt awkward, like I was often in the way. It was hard to keep up with my obstetrics resident dashing around the labor and delivery area. I tried to play man-to-man defense and stay close to him as he zipped around. One time I realized I had followed him into the bathroom. Embarrassing.

That first morning, the increasing moans of a woman in labor beckoned me to the delivery room. "Don't drop the baby, don't drop the baby," I chanted quietly to myself.

Then it was go-time. The resident slapped the scissors in my palm and looked into my eyes, "As soon as you see the umbilical cord, you cut it!"

I perked up. I had my orders. Exhausted and trembling with scissors in hand, I blocked out everything I had read about childbirth so I could focus on my one job. As I stood there waiting, I had a flashback to when I was a teenager, working as a volunteer firefighter back in Danville, Pennsylvania, holding an empty hose that began to vibrate as the water turned on. "There it is, *CUT IT!*" my resident yelled as the baby's cord emerged and they put clamps on it. I swooped in and cut it in about 1.5 seconds. I nailed it.

But before I could celebrate, I noticed how suddenly the pulsations in the cord stopped. I had cut off blood flow from the mom to the baby. For some reason, it felt a little wrong. *Oh well,* I thought, *that seemed weird, but I guess the baby has to disconnect eventually.* But, what happened next seemed even more unnatural. The mom reached out to hold her newborn, as if it were a natural reflex, but my resident immediately whisked the baby away. In the back area of the room, he gave *me* the baby to hold. I wrapped myself around this tiny kid in a quasi bear hug to ensure I didn't drop him.

"What now?" I asked my resident.

"We have to work on the baby," he replied.

Work on him? I was curious what he meant.

He looked at the cute baby and said, "Welcome to the world," placing the baby on a table. The first task was to measure the "reflex irritability score" by irritating the child — part of the Apgar assessment routinely done in the last 60 years.[1] My most vivid memory is of my resident inserting a metal temperature probe into the baby's rectum. I got along well with this resident, so I felt comfortable speaking my mind. "Now that doesn't seem like a nice way to welcome a new human to the world," I told him.

"We have to get the baby's temperature . . . and to make sure the rectum is open," he replied.

"Why?" I asked.

"To record the temperature on the sheet as we rewarm the baby. Newborns get cold quickly."

I looked at this crying baby under a French-fry heat lamp with a metal temperature probe in his butt. It just seemed wrong. (Thankfully, these days temperature is measured noninvasively.) It was also ironic. The baby could have stayed warm in the arms of his mother, who was so hot she was sweating. I also wondered (as I frequently did as a student) if I had made things worse. I had cut off a direct transfusion of warm blood to the baby with my rapid snip of the umbilical cord.

The White Coat Era

For most of human history, moms held their newborns upon delivery. Because the umbilical cord was not immediately cut, babies received a boost of oxygenated blood for the first few minutes of life as they transitioned to breathing air. They were also kept warm in Mama's arms, where they were more likely to latch and breast-feed. But then doctors became an elevated class in the post–World War era. They began wearing white coats and had the ability to prescribe antibiotics that could instantly cure people. Surgery went from being barbaric and painful to safe and controlled. Hospitals became revered sanctuaries, housing new medical technology that mesmerized the public. Doctors went from using a lancet and bandages to complex incubators and iron lung machines. The authority of doctors soared. A new medical culture emerged. Doctors took the liberty of holding people in the hospital for prolonged periods for observation and testing.

This new culture profoundly changed the way we treated babies. By the 1950s any healthy baby was separated from its mother at birth and held in the hospital for seven days. Doctors confined all newborns to one room to make it easier to round on them. Occasionally, parents could peer through a glass window to see their child's crib in a sea of babies. Many babies were formula-fed while they were being detained and some had no sense of night or day because the fluorescent lights were always on. By the 1970s, the hospital stay for a healthy full-term baby had drifted down to three days. Parents who asked to hold their babies in the hospital were warned of health risks and told to wait until the doctor "cleared" the baby. I remember when my sister was born perfectly normal and "at term" in the 1980s. After Mom came home, we asked when our new sister was coming home from the hospital. The next day, the doctors "released" her.

Premature babies had a much tougher go.[2] Most got strapped down and intubated. That is, they had breathing tubes inserted down their throats and were attached to a ventilator. Many were given 100% oxygen, which was later found to cause blindness[3] and even leukemia.[4] Some babies born premature did not have difficulty breathing, but they were nevertheless intubated and given high levels of oxygen as a part of a protocol.

Pediatricians and obstetricians were taught that premature babies had nerves too underdeveloped to feel pain.[5] Even major operations were done on preemies without anesthesia, a practice that continued into the 1970s. Preemies were medically paralyzed during surgery but given nothing for pain. In other words, they couldn't move but they were awake during procedures and could feel everything.

A similarly bizarre and brutal practice was to withhold all food, water, or glucose from a premature baby. The dogma was first popularized by Dr. Julius Hess, who began the first U.S. center for premature infants at Michael Reese Hospital in Chicago. Hess wrote in his widely read 1941 textbook, "It has been our experience that too early feeding may often be the cause of aspiration pneumonia and is, therefore, to be avoided." He recommended instead that "the premature baby receives physiologic salt solution, subcutaneously in the thighs, one to three times daily."[6]

In other words, nothing by mouth, but we'll stick your baby with a needle in the thigh. Starving preemies to death persisted until the late 1960s. One dissenting pediatrician challenged the prevailing dogma by presenting data that starving premature babies increased mortality by 70%.[7] But his study was largely ignored. It's shocking, but the hospital practice of starving babies to death in the name of health continued for decades.[8] (As an aside, similar dogma about not allowing women in labor to eat or drink lingers to this day, despite a 2013 study that found "no justification for the restriction of fluids and food" in low-risk women.)[9] Eventually the risk of aspiration from feeding babies was debunked. Isolating, starving, and injecting preemies with saltwater in any other setting would be prosecuted today. Looking back, it was assault and neglect.

Touched by an Angel

I felt rattled by what I read in old pediatric textbooks and articles. At times, I felt like I was watching a horror movie, and I wasn't allowed to close my eyes. Other times, I was in awe of some of my predecessors. There were good doctors who treated babies as precious humans and discovered good interventions that saved lives. One of those doctors was Dr. Marilee Allen, a now-retired Johns Hopkins neonatologist who was practicing at the time. I reached out to her to learn more about the culture of the era.

"People thought babies couldn't feel pain," she told me. "I never believed it."

I asked her what had caused her to question conventional thinking at the time. "I had a good teacher who taught me to *think,*" she told me. Dr. Allen explained that while newborns are not able to tell you they are in pain, you could see pain in their vitals. Their heart rate and blood pressure shot up during procedures and they would often swat at any instrument that prodded them.

I remember seeing this during circumcisions. As a medical student, I watched little baby boys strapped to a plastic board before having their penis foreskin cut, with nothing given for pain, as they writhed in attempts to escape. One little guy turned blue as he was screaming. It looked sadistic. Afterward, the tiny boys were jittery with diaper changes. One stopped breast-feeding for a day after the traumatic procedure, which my resident told me was common.

"He won't remember it," he told me.

"What does that have to do with anything?" I replied. "Are we worried he was going to recount the feeling to a jury someday?" My resident didn't seem happy with my questions and sent me to the cafeteria to get the team food. Remarkably, another baby boy who had a circumcision later that week seemed to feel no pain. I had more pain from watching.

I recounted these observations to Dr. Allen. "Your instincts were good, Marty," she replied. We should always use some anesthetic, she explained.

From time to time during her career as a busy neonatologist, Dr. Allen would take a step back from the rush of saving lives to ponder what the medical culture was doing. Separating babies from their moms was the norm. Sticking them in the heel to draw blood — one, two, or three times a day — was standard operating procedure. Doing these things day in and day out compelled her to look at the big picture. "This is so harsh. This is not nurturing," she told me. Of course, sometimes this care was necessary to save lives. But, as she acknowledged, her generation of doctors often didn't know what was best for the baby.

I was impressed by Dr. Allen's passion for defenseless children. Hours into our conversation, I learned that she'd had a premature son herself in the 1980s. The first time she laid eyes on him in the NICU, about 24 hours after his birth, she cried and apologized to him. She knew her tears were not rational because she had done nothing wrong. But for the first time, she felt the intense bond between mother and child and could sense his suffering. "Mothers carry guilt when they have a premature baby. We have to nurture them through it," she said.

Our conversation about her long career at Johns Hopkins and the medical dogma of the field seemed therapeutic for her. Then she shared something shocking, something other older neonatologists had also hinted at. When a baby was born stillborn, or alive but considered nonviable, doctors had whisked it away so the mom couldn't see its face.

"They tried to prevent moms from seeing the baby," she told me, offering this meager explanation: "It was to protect the mom and the staff from the drama." The doctors had thought it would be bad for a grieving mom to see her baby. "We didn't understand grieving," she added. It was a form of medical paternalism.

Dr. Allen had felt strongly that in the mechanical quest to save premature babies, their caregivers were forgetting to nurture them. It had led her to launch an initiative that allowed a dedicated team of people to nurture each baby born at Johns Hopkins. To cuddle and love them. Sometimes they could hold a baby, other times they extended a pinky for a little baby hand to grip. She called it the NEST team (Nurturing

Environment Support Team), and it continues at Johns Hopkins to this day. She also made every attempt to have mothers hold their babies, even when the baby was on a respirator. It was hard, and not always possible, but when safety precautions could be taken, this contact provided a powerful dose of healing.

Closet Babies

One extreme manifestation of the paternalism of medicine was the practice of putting a premature infant, on the border of viability, in a closet to die. I'm not referring to an isolated case of some twisted murder mystery that was featured on the true crime show *Dateline*. This occurred at some hospitals for decades. That's right: Doctors would routinely take living premature babies (typically less than 27 weeks gestational age) and leave them somewhere to die. Some neonatologists told me that this practice lingered until the 1990s. After doctors told parents that their baby could not survive, they'd put the baby in some kind of open container and stash them in a closet. One neonatologist explained to me that closets prevented the staff from having to hear the baby's anguished cries.

Dr. Dan Hermann is a physician in Bedminster, New Jersey. He was born in 1968 as a premature baby at 28 weeks gestational age. He was likely one of those babies left to die. His mother was not given all the details, but what Hermann knows is that he was born on the border of viability and was not initially treated with full resuscitative measures — as would be expected if you wanted a child to live. After some time, however, given his persistent signs of life, doctors decided to do everything to try to save him with the full-court press.

They inserted a breathing tube and administered high levels of oxygen, ignoring evidence that high oxygen causes blindness in preemies. Dan survived and grew up to enroll at Johns Hopkins and eventually became a pediatrician. In residency, he was considered by his fellow residents to be one of the smartest and most compassionate doctors they had ever known. His thick glasses are the only residual effect of his birth saga. He needs them because his eyes were damaged by the excessive oxygen. Herman had four operations on his eyes, including a cataract operation before his residency. Today he can only see out of one of his eyes and in two dimensions.

"My parents named me Daniel because of Daniel in the lion's den," he told me with a smile.

For years, Dr. Hermann has shared his personal story to teach and inspire young doctors and students about the value of human life. One of the junior residents he inspired was a young doctor from India, Arpi Chiruvolu, who dedicated her life to newborn care because of his mentorship. She went on to conduct groundbreaking scientific research that weaves together the sophistication of modern medicine with the ancient craft of newborn care.

A Fresh Perspective

Dr. Arpitha Chiruvolu grew up in Hyderabad, India, where she also went to medical school. As a student rotating in the neonatal ICU in India, she witnessed a premature baby that had an extremely poor prognosis. The mom held the baby on her chest and sang to him for days, breast-feeding him with a touch of milk from time to time. To her surprise, the baby developed normally without any neurological problems. This made a big impression on Dr. Chiruvolu.

She was struck by the medicalization of childbirth when she came to the U.S. in the early 2000s. The rapid cord-cutting, heat lamps, formula feeding, and the practice of separating babies from Mama were standard. In India, they didn't have enough hospital cribs for babies. They taught husbands to support the mothers so they could safely hold the baby skin-to-skin for at least six hours a day. They encouraged early breast-feeding and kept babies and mothers together, so moms had easy access to cradle and cuddle their newborns.

Inspired by Dr. Hermann, she became a neonatologist at Baylor University Medical Center. In my research for this book, she came highly recommended to me as a true pioneer in the field. In fact, doctors around the country told me I should check out what this doctor in Texas was doing and read her studies. I reached out to her and traveled to McKinney, Texas, to spend a day learning from her. What I witnessed blew me away.

A genteel and unassuming woman, Dr. Chiruvolu greeted me and escorted me to her office. We got acquainted over a cup of coffee, and then she put her hand on a folder full of research articles she had printed for me. "There are many modern discoveries in newborn care," she explained. "The biggest one is that we need to decrease the level of medical interventions. Allow the baby to be a baby."

Dr. Chiruvolu's passion stemmed from observing medicine in India and the U.S., and from reading studies about U.S. obstetricians in the 1960s and '70s who challenged the status quo at the time. She took a particular interest in emerging U.S. approaches to newborn care that mimicked what had been standard of care in India. These "new" U.S. approaches included:

- Delayed cord clamping
- Holding the baby skin-to-skin with the mother
- Breast-feeding in the first hour
- Giving preemies a minute to breathe before intervening
- Using antibiotics *selectively* to treat infections, not routinely
- Avoiding C-section unless medically necessary

But whether a mom and baby in her Texas hospital received these best practices depended on which doctor happened to be on call. Dr. Chiruvolu implemented a protocol at the Baylor Scott and White health care system to standardize care. She also collected outcomes data to measure their impact.

Nature's Boost

I recounted to Dr. Chiruvolu how I had cut umbilical cords immediately as a medical student. She shook her head and smiled. She explained that the blood pumped to a baby in the first few minutes outside the womb is not just any blood. It's rich in stem cells, fetal hemoglobin (which boosts the transfer of oxygen), nutrients, and antibodies to boost immunity. Years of standardizing delayed cord clamping at her hospital had demonstrated to her that babies were less likely to then need intravenous fluids or to develop infections.

The benefits of the extra blood a baby gets through delayed cord clamping were magnified with premature babies. Those who had delayed cord clamping were far less likely to require a blood transfusion,[10,11] less likely to require ventilation,[12] less likely to require medication to increase their blood pressure (aka vasopressors), less likely to be admitted to a neonatal ICU,[13] and had shorter hospital stays. She published many of these results in the medical literature. Her studies also demonstrated a benefit of delayed cord clamping in C-section births.[14] To show just how valuable the cord could be, she published a study that showed delaying the clamping by 60 seconds after birth resulted in better outcomes compared to clamping the cord after 45 seconds, suggesting that every little bit seems to help.[15] Since my time with her, a clinical trial showed that waiting 2 minutes is better than 30 seconds.[16] In 2023, a different study from Australia suggested that delayed cord clamping could halve the risk of death in preemies.[17,18] If any pill did that, we'd say every mother should take it.

Dr. Chiruvolu marveled at the simplicity of this important aspect of the delivery. "This is such an amazing intervention that has been ignored for decades because doctors wanted to quickly get babies to their examination area. The benefits to delayed cord clamping have been known for a long time, but it was ignored because we wanted to get our stuff done. It's also amazing that this intervention doesn't cost a penny."

There may also be long-term benefits. Dr. Chiruvolu pointed me to a little-known 2022 study that had found that delayed cord clamping may help a baby's brain development. Researchers performed MRIs on babies when they reached age one and reported that infants who had been afforded delayed cord clamping "had greater myelin content in important brain regions involved in motor function, visual/spatial, and sensory processing."[19] Amazing.

"How often is delayed cord clamping done?" I asked Dr. Chiruvolu.

"There has been a shift in the last decade,"

she replied. “It’s now done in approximately 90% of U.S. births, but it’s also important to do it the right way.” She explained that it’s good to give the cord at least a minute — or wait until it stops pulsating or turns white. She often has mothers hold their baby on their chest while the cord is still pulsating. It’s not an absolute rule, she pointed out, because some babies need emergent resuscitation and must have their cords cut right away.

My Nephew

When I watched my nephew being born about ten years ago, doctors immediately cut the cord and whisked him away to intensive care for two days. My sister didn’t see him for those two days. I asked why he was being taken to the NICU, and they said he was having “difficulty transitioning.” I asked what they meant by that, and they told me it encompassed several things: a slightly elevated heart rate, some irregular breathing, and a bilirubin level that was a bit high.

When I got the actual bilirubin level, I pointed out that it was only borderline, not high, and that the best therapy for his “difficulty transitioning” was to get him in the arms of his mother. In my opinion, the reason he was having this "transitioning" problem is that they pumped my sister with oxytocin to induce labor. The medication likely increased the rate of his little heart.

My nephew had trouble breast-feeding for a long time, which I believe may have been aggravated by the over-medicalization of his birth. I shared these observations with Dr. Chiruvolu, who told me that children separated at birth for days can indeed have trouble latching and breast-feeding, due to the prolonged separation. She also told me that what happened to my nephew has been common in the U.S. "The best place to transition is on the mother's chest, skin-to-skin, for the vast majority of babies," she said. She added that this point has been lost over the past several decades of relying on medical technology.

Keep Moms and Babies Together

When Dr. Chiruvolu became the chief of her hospital's neonatal ICU, she wanted to end the routine practice of separating newborns from their mothers. In 2012, she introduced a new process. She had a crib for newborns placed in each mother's hospital room (which made it more tedious for doctors to round on the babies, but easier for the moms to hold and feed them). Some doctors didn't like the new arrangement. One doctor even complained to her, "Is this Africa?"

"Africa has good things to teach us, we need to learn from Africa," she replied.

Years later, that same doctor told her that he loved the new system.

There's something magical about the *bonding* between a newborn and mother. Dr. Chiruvolu and I spoke about how we don't fully understand it, and we can't entirely measure it in medicine, but it's powerful.

Modern medicine's rediscovery of the benefits of skin-to-skin contact began after a village nurse in Colombia suggested the idea to two pediatricians in Bogotá in the 1970s. The pediatricians, Drs. Edgar Rey and Héctor Martínez, liked the idea (especially given the shortage of incubators) and began incorporating it in their care of premature babies. They soon witnessed a 70% decrease in deaths with the skin-to-skin technique.[20] They likened the technique to the female gray kangaroo, which gives birth to tiny babies and keeps them in her pouch as a natural incubator. This simple technique saved lives, but many doctors were insulted by the idea. Scathing commentaries (with no hard data) attempted to discredit them, including a *Lancet* article titled "Myth of the Marsupial Mother."[21]

Years later, a Swedish missionary doctor working in Zimbabwe, Dr. Nils Bergman, made another attempt to propose the idea in the medical literature. He felt it was unnatural to separate babies from their moms at birth as modern medicine demanded at the time. In 1994 he authored an article on the "kangaroo-method" for treating low-birth-weight babies.[22] Western doctors in the medical establishment lambasted Dr. Bergman for his backward approach while boasting of their neonatal incubators and technological might. The debate continued for decades, with minimal adoption of the skin-to-skin protocol in the U.S.

Throughout her career Dr. Chiruvolu was convinced of the benefits of skin-to-skin time based on the scientific data, her own bedside observations, and her intuition. But the protocol had not been widely adopted throughout her hospital and its affiliates. So in 2015, she implemented a policy for all newborns to be held by their mothers skin-to-skin for 2 to 12 hours, when safe and feasible. Fathers were also taught to hold the baby skin-to-skin. The longer the better, but an exhausted mother may need help to ensure she can safely hold a baby when she's sleep-deprived, the doctor explained to me.

The results were incredible: a 25% increase in breast-feeding,[23] a 50% reduction in babies going to the NICU, and a 50% reduction in postpartum depression.[24] Holding a baby may be a mother's best antidepressant drug. Dr. Chiruvolu also showed me data that newborns held with prolonged skin-to-skin time had a more normal heartrate, blood pressure, and even blood glucose levels.[25,26]

"Wait a minute," I interjected. I told her I could see how skin-to-skin time can result in a baby having a more normal heart rate and blood pressure. But blood glucose level? I didn't understand what the mechanism would be there.

"The baby's stress hormones are not spiking as high when the mom holds the baby, and stress hormones [what we call corticosteroids] increase blood glucose levels, a fight-or-flight stress response," Dr. Chiruvolu explained.

Ah, of course, that made sense. My first thought was about my poor little nephew. He had likely been experiencing higher than necessary spikes in his stress hormones after being separated from his mother at birth.

Dr. Chiruvolu published her findings, and national medical organizations began to take note. Her 2017 study showing that prolonged skin-to-skin time helps control a baby's blood sugar level was incorporated into national guidelines of the Academy of Breastfeeding Medicine. And in 2023, the WHO issued a broad recommendation for small and pre-term babies to have skin-to-skin contact with their mother for 8 to 12 hours a day, starting immediately after birth.[27] To this day, some hospitals refer to the skin-to-skin technique as "kangaroo care."

Dr. Chiruvolu is not just a sharp neonatologist who is skilled at delivering advanced medical care for sick newborns. She also believes in making medical care more humane. When the baby must be in a neonatal ICU, she will apply all the might of modern medicine to save a child or prevent disability. But amid the rush of delivering high-level care, she also pauses to have the mom safely hold the baby, skin-to-skin, even while the baby is on a ventilator.

"Prematurity is not a sickness," Dr. Chiruvolu told me. "They are just early. They deserve breast milk and to be with their mother."

Microbiome Alert

For most of the modern era, doctors have routinely given every premature baby antibiotics, a practice that sadly lingers to this day. Retired University of Wisconsin neonatologist Dr. Frank Greer told me that back when he was a resident in the 1970s, antibiotics were commonly overprescribed because doctors — as we've seen — thought they had no downsides. Antibiotic use was so excessive that most times when he tested a baby's poop looking for gastrointestinal infection, the lab report showed zero bacteria. In other words, preemies were so pumped with antibiotics they produced sterile poop.

Dr. Chiruvolu also recalled lab reports showing bacteria-free poop from when she was a resident. Other neonatologists I spoke to all said they had witnessed the same thing — sterile shit.

I asked Dr. Chiruvolu how often a premature baby truly requires an antibiotic. "Rarely," she said. "There should be a reason to give it." For example, some newborns can get dangerously sick from a bacterial infection of the placenta. In these cases, it's critical to start an antibiotic promptly. But the blanket use of antibiotics in all premature babies can harm some children by altering their microbiome precisely when it begins to take form. One *JAMA* study published in 2018 found that 94% of premature babies are given antibiotics, even though only about 10 to 20% truly need them for a suspected infection.[28] Equally disturbing, when test results came back showing that a newborn did not have an infection, more than half of the babies were kept on antibiotics for another half a week or more. After studying the microbiome, I was apoplectic when I read the recent stats about the number of babies who are having their microbiome affected by antibiotics. We saw similar types of nonsensical prescribing during the opioid epidemic. We have a crisis of appropriateness.

Dr. Chiruvolu is a big believer in the importance of the microbiome. Antibiotics can save lives, but they also alter the microbiome. That's why she teaches to stop antibiotics as soon as test results show they're no longer needed. As I've seen in my own specialty, stopping antibiotics tends to be an afterthought, and as a result, many patients stay on them far longer than they need to. "We're trying so hard to promote a healthy microbiome in our babies," she told me.

Her philosophy is also the basis of a protocol she implemented to ensure that babies are fed colostrum, which is the nutrient-rich milk a mom initially produces. At her hospital, they encourage breast-feeding in the first "golden hour" of life. If a baby has to be separated for medical reasons, a team will ask the mother to provide her colostrum in a syringe so they can use it in the neonatal ICU to seed the baby's microbiome.

Dr. Chiruvolu has also resurrected the practice of not bathing a healthy newborn for a day, and a preemie for a week. That may sound kind of gross. Why does she recommend it? A baby is covered with a protein layer of amniotic fluid that helps retain its body heat and carries bacteria that seed a healthy microbiome. To help promote this healthy seeding of the microbiome, some hospitals are taking this idea a step further. They are studying the potential benefit of swabbing the skin of newborns born by C-section with vaginal fluid (assuming the woman does not have an infection like HPV or gonorrhea).[29]

As a medical student, one of my jobs was to wash newborn babies so we could check the boxes on our chart and hand the mom a shiny new baby. I had no idea that in doing so, I was washing away a layer of fluid that could keep the baby warm and promote a healthy microbiome.

Measuring Appropriateness

Some hospitals are now collecting data on how they perform on some of the best practices presented in this chapter. Some newborns

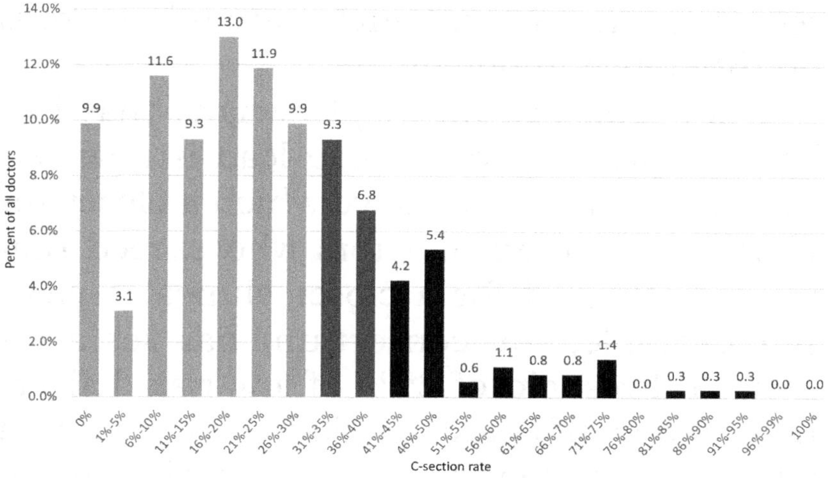

*Distribution of physicians by their C-section rates in low-risk deliveries.**

(Dr. Will Bruhn, Global Appropriateness Measures. *Data of 354 New York State physicians who deliver low-risk babies at a high volume.)

need antibiotics, but not all of them. Some children should be whisked away for critical resuscitation, but not all of them. And some babies should be delivered by C-section — but not all of them. Rates of intervention should vary, but within certain boundaries. In the case of C-section, they are medically necessary in approximately 10 to 15% of pregnancies, according to the WHO, yet the rate is double that in some U.S. hospitals. The statistic exceeds 50% in some parts of the world, such as Brazil.[30] In many other countries, nearly all deliveries in private hospitals are by C-section. That was my observation on a recent trip to Egypt. Patients are told there is no difference in outcomes.

A new consortium of physicians that I've had the privilege of helping lead is now setting threshold rates, above which a closer review is warranted. Doctors who exceed that rate are flagged for a closer clinical review. For example, the consortium has set a C-section threshold of 25% of low-risk deliveries in a doctor's practice. Any doctor with an annual C–section rate over 25% is flagged for a closer review of their individual C-section cases by their peers. Exceptions are made for doctors who staff midwifery deliveries and are only called in to perform C-sections. We identified doctors with C-section rates ranging from 0 to more than 90%. We shared the following distribution of OB doctors' C-section rates in New York State with the governor's lead health-care officers.[31]

Precise data like this can drive up the quality of health care while reducing harmful and costly waste. Our consortium, called Global Appropriateness Measures (GAM), has created hundreds of similar measures looking at practice patterns across 40 medical specialties. (You can learn more about the effort at www.gameasures.com.)

Medical schools do many things well. Teaching the appropriateness of care is not one of them. Traditional quality measures only examine what's already been done by doctors. They do not capture whether a given medical intervention was necessary. As a result, we develop blind spots in medicine, areas of overuse where alarming practice patterns go undetected.

What began as an idea to measure appropriateness — an idea I introduced in my book *The Price We Pay* — has emerged as a new dimension of physician quality used throughout health care. Hundreds of appropriateness measures are now being applied, using big data to screen for extreme-outlier physician practice patterns. This information is being used today by hospitals for internal quality improvement, as well as by primary care practices and patient navigators who then steer people to doctors who perform well on the appropriateness of their care. The big dilemma emerging in health care today: Now that we can measure appropriateness of care with robust measures, do we have a moral duty to look at the data? I believe we do.

Once a C-Section, Always a C-Section?

A common dogma that prevails in obstetrics today is the rule that if you had a C-section, all future births must be by C-section. It was popularized in the 1990s, heavily influenced by newspaper headlines attributing uterine rupture (which is extremely rare) to vaginal delivery after C-section. In some cases, the dictum conveniently justified the preference of the obstetrician or the mother to *schedule* a C-section. (Staying up all night as an obstetrician taking periodic catnaps can be miserable.) By 2006, the once-a-C-section-always-a-C-section dogma dominated the field of obstetrics as well as public opinion. A study that year found that fewer than 1% of women had a vaginal birth after C-section (VBAC).[32] But today there is a renewed appreciation of the benefits of attempting to have a vaginal delivery when it can be safely performed. In fact, one obstetrician I know just delivered a woman's eighth consecutive child vaginally after the first child was born by C-section.

In 2014, the *Wall Street Journal* printed a story about a mother who wanted a VBAC. Her hospital had a policy not to do them. She found another hospital willing to evaluate her and try and, sure enough, she was able to deliver her second child vaginally. This story increased public skepticism about the rule.

To better understand this issue, I reached

out to Dr. Leslie Hansen Lindner. I first met her as a medical student on my OB/GYN rotation. Her passion to always put patients first stood out — no matter the hour or the patient's income or insurance status. There is no one I trust more to deliver a baby. When I was a medical student, I witnessed her take command of surgical emergencies, empathize with patients to comfort them, and quote research studies to them with greater recall than ChatGPT. For every issue in the field, I watched her objectively present all options, and then weigh in with her recommendation when she had one — a style I try to emulate in my practice to this day. Just to show you how sharp she was, Dr. Hansen Lindner immediately called out the leaders of the Women's Health Initiative study, who I wrote about in chapter 2, "OMG HRT," when they falsely claimed that hormone replacement therapy causes breast cancer.

Dr. Hansen Lindner is now a busy obstetrician gynecologist in Charlotte, North Carolina, where she is chief of OB/GYN at Atrium Health and chair of the quality committee. I called her to ask her if it was really true that once a woman had a C-section, she always needed a C-section.

"That's not true," she replied. "Marty, my VBAC success rate is about 80%." This, despite the fact that many of her patients are considered high-risk. Nationally the VBAC success rate is 60 to 80% when women opt to try.[33]

The move back to VBAC got a boost in 2006 when an NIH monograph reminded doctors and the public alike that there are many factors that should go into the decision, not just a myopic fear of uterine rupture. A group of obstetricians also set up an online VBAC calculator that has helped women understand that the once-a-C-section mantra was not an absolute rooted in science, as many people think.[34]

Does Every Woman Need to Be Induced?

"There's one more thing you should look at," Dr. Hansen Lindner told me as we started to wrap up our meeting. "You should have your research team at Hopkins take a look at the ARRIVE trial."

Ah yes, I recalled the ARRIVE trial. The landmark 2018 study counterintuitively made inducing labor a new standard of care for nearly every low-risk pregnancy, as opposed to using it on occasion, only when deemed necessary.[35]

The study enrolled approximately 6,000 women with low-risk pregnancies and randomized them when they got to 38 weeks. Half were given a drug like Pitocin to induce labor at 39 weeks, and the other half were treated "expectantly," that is, doctors waited for the woman to go into labor on her own (with some exceptions), as doctors had been doing for centuries. The study, published in the *New England Journal,* claimed that the routine induction of labor group suffered fewer complications. But oddly, the study made its claim of superiority by adding unrelated outcomes together — outcomes that were not statistically significant by themselves. They also skewed their results by bizarrely allowing expectant mothers to progress far longer in their pregnancy than most obstetricians would feel comfortable because of the known harms of delivering after 42 weeks. The study design seemed stacked against waiting for labor to occur naturally.

I printed out the study and handed it to our research team to examine its methodology. The two statisticians at the meeting quickly pointed out the same problem: grouping compilations into "bundles." Grouping rare events is a well-known way to "massage the results," to take a study that does not show a statistically significant difference and make it show one. Our research team concluded that the study had major limitations, some of which the authors even acknowledged in their article. The team felt that the *New England Journal* should have rejected the study.

Despite the study's design flaws, it changed practices in America. Beginning in 2018, some hospitals instituted routine induction for all low-risk women at 39 weeks, in part because of the ARRIVE trial. Dr. Hansen Lindner and many other doctors, however, have not changed the way they practice.

A subsequent study published in 2023 pointed out that since the publication of the ARRIVE trial, the number of inductions had gone up, but with no reduction in complication rates, countering the predictions of the ARRIVE authors.[36] If a repeat study contradicts the ARRIVE study, it would not be the first time that a current practice based on a *New England Journal* study got reversed. For most of the last two decades, the drug Makena was hailed as the first medication that could prevent preterm labor, which leads to premature newborns. For centuries, nothing has worked to stop this problem. The drug received an accelerated FDA approval in 2011 based on a *New England Journal* study[37] and was given to more than a quarter million women, many of them poor and on Medicaid. But then scientists at the FDA pointed out a critical flaw in the study, and a better study published in 2021 found the drug was no different from placebo in preventing preterm labor. In other words, it didn't work. Two and a half years later the FDA pulled it off the market. (Why it took them two and a half years to do so is another story, about the FDA's bureaucracy.)[38]

When my friend was looking for an obstetrician to deliver her baby, she took my suggestion to ask prospective doctors if they routinely induce all low-risk pregnancies at 39 weeks. One obstetrician said "yes," and robotically cited the ARRIVE trial results like a catechism. Another she spoke to presented a nuanced answer expressing some concerns about the ARRIVE study. I told her to go with the latter obstetrician.

Humility

Advanced medicine can save the life of a newborn. But many of modern medicine's common rituals performed on newborns have not been based on scientific evidence. They have instead been dictated by medical dogma. Some fly directly in the face of both science and wisdom.

Take, for example, the practice I mentioned

earlier of giving newborn babies in distress 100% oxygen (as opposed to room air). That this caused blindness was established in 1952 by the head of ophthalmology at Johns Hopkins, Dr. Arnall Patz, who was awarded the Presidential Medal of Freedom for the discovery. He dared to challenge conventional wisdom that oxygen is all good. He used science to question the assumption that what is good for an adult must also be good for a child.

Yet for many years the harmful practice continued to be propagated by the American Academy of Pediatrics through its Neonatal Resuscitation Program course. It wasn't until 2005 that the guidelines changed for full-term babies. Premature babies would have to wait until 2010 for the guidelines to give doctors the discretion to give between 21 and 100% oxygen, and by 2015, guidelines changed to recommend 21 to 30% oxygen to resuscitate premature babies.

I asked Dr. Hermann, who had sustained eye damage from the high oxygen he was given as a preemie, how he felt about the medical profession taking 63 years to fully implement findings of Dr. Patz from 1952.

"I think it's incredible. I could have had vision in both eyes . . . because we knew about it."

A Pendulum

The story of modern childbirth shows how the pendulum swings from one extreme to the other.

Doctors who decades ago insisted on keeping newborns in the hospital for seven days were not mad scientists hell-bent on holding newborns in captivity like captured aliens. They were responding to a bygone era when childbirth had been extremely dangerous. In 1915, the first year that infant mortality rates were recorded, 10% of all newborns in the U.S. died.[39] Demanding that mothers and babies stay in the controlled setting of a hospital was an emergency measure to address the havoc. It was also an opportunity to study newborns. The medical establishment began to learn and standardized the resuscitation of babies. Today infant mortality is 93% lower than what it had been.

But at the same time, the medical field has developed large blind spots.

It's rare for the pendulum of appropriate care to stay in the center, where we want it. In other words, finding the perfect balance of just the right amount of medical care and the right amount of nature is hard. Sadly, the pendulum tends to make big swings.

If we are being honest with the numbers, infant mortality declined steeply over time, despite the many errors of past generations of doctors. But the pendulum has swung too far in the direction of over-medicalization. Today thousands of parents, turned off by cold medical practices of the past and present, have soured on modern medicine and don't want to have anything to do with it. They sometimes glamorize home births and medical-free deliveries, ignoring the real risks such decisions entail. Yes, a home birth is more intervention-free, and less expensive when everything goes well. But home deliveries triple the risk of infant mortality.

The answer isn't to swing the pendulum far to one side or the other. We must avoid reactionary extremes. In every area of medicine, we should ask ourselves where we are in the pendulum swing. Can we avoid overtreatment, and what blind spots have we developed?

Modern medicine saves lives, but we also need to ensure it restores humane practices to childbirth, the world's most ancient medical procedure.

CHAPTER 8

CHALLENGING CERTAINTY

The true origin of ovarian cancer

Uncertainty is an uncomfortable position. But certainty is an absurd one.

— Voltaire

Over his 30-year career, Dr. B hated breaking bad news to women that they had ovarian cancer. It's often incurable by the time it's discovered, and as a result, it's the most fatal gynecologic cancer in the world.[1] Even more discouraging, there is no effective screening test for it.[2]

Dr. B is an empathetic guy. He tends to get emotionally connected to his patients. With each passing year, he became angrier at ovarian cancer. It got to the point where he actually got angry at the ovaries themselves! From his jaded vantage point, it didn't matter that the ovary produces healthy hormones. In his mind, the ovary served no purpose except to terrorize women when a cancer grew out of it. Occasionally in the operating room, the surgical dissection would reveal the gleaming organ in plain sight. He would pause and stare it down, like a soldier staring his enemy in the eyes.

Dr. B was on a mission to convince every woman of post-childbearing age that needed surgery for any reason to also have her ovaries removed to prevent cancer. Throughout his career, Dr. B took out thousands.

His view was not far off from the norm over the last 70 years. My colleague Dr. Rebecca Stone, chief of gynecologic oncology at Johns Hopkins, told me she felt the same way for much of her career. But as a woman, she had more mixed emotions. She told me she felt sad that an organ that is so important for everything from our sex drive to temperature regulation can kill so viciously. Many gynecology surgeons told me the same thing. Nationwide, hundreds of millions of perfectly normal ovaries have been, and continue to be, removed in the name of cancer prevention.

The crusade to remove normal ovaries to save lives seemed to be going great until a dramatic and humbling discovery was recently made: Ovarian cancer does not come from the ovary.

Doctors were targeting the wrong organ.

"What?" I thought, as Dr. Stone explained

this new research finding to me one afternoon at the hospital. I had to stop her several times. "You mean to tell me that ovarian cancer does not come from the ovary?"

That's right, she explained. According to new research, the most common type of ovarian cancer, serous cancer, originates from the fallopian tube.

"But the name of the disease is *ovarian* cancer. How can it be that it doesn't come from the ovary?" She told me new research was shedding light on a centuries-long assumption.

I was flabbergasted. Could this really be true? And if it was, how had I not learned about this sooner? Later that day, I called physician friends from around the country to see if they had heard of this mind-bending discovery. Most had not. I decided to hunt down all the research on this topic and take a deep dive. I plunged into some of the most startling, most fascinating research I've seen in the last decade. It was an intellectual whiplash with serious implications for millions of women.

Scientific Courage

In 1999, Dr. Louis Dubeau, a University of Southern California pathologist, wrote an essay floating the radical idea. He had observed that some ovarian cancer cells didn't seem to have the features of ovary cells.[3] The title of his highly controversial article asked, "Does the Emperor Have No Clothes?" It turns out the answer was yes.

In 2001, a group of Dutch pathologists were puzzled while examining the ovaries of women who'd had them removed because they were considered high-risk for ovarian cancer. The pathologists found budding pre-cancer cells — but not in the ovary. They were millimeters away in the fallopian tube, both of which were removed at the same time.[4]

At the Dana-Farber Cancer Institute, pathologist Dr. Christopher Crum heard about these counterintuitive findings of the Dutch group. "I don't believe them," he initially thought. But his mentor encouraged him to be unbiased and test the hypothesis. So he conducted a more extensive study and, lo and behold, found that serous cancer comes from the fallopian tube.[5] Specifically, from a part called the fimbriae, the finger-like projections at the end of the tube that drape over the ovary. I reached out to Dr. Crum and spoke with him about his study, which came out in 2006. He explained that at first many scientists in the field did not accept his research. In fact, his first article was rejected for publication because the reviewers, who seemed confused by the results, thought the idea was too far-fetched. One rejection letter stated, "The authors propose a theory that is interesting but also requires significant imagination."

But that was precisely the point of his study. The rejection letter suggested that ovarian cancer couldn't possibly come from the fallopian tube because it came from the ovary, missing the discovery altogether.

"I've got colleagues who have really hung on to the ovarian origin idea, but you have to keep an open mind," Dr. Crum told me. "You have to be willing to evolve your thinking."

Then in 2017, my colleague Dr. Victor Velculescu further settled the tubal origin debate with an elegant study.[6] A professor of pathology and oncology at Johns Hopkins, he collaborated with University of Pennsylvania researcher Dr. Ronnie Drapkin, who trained under Dr. Crum. Together, they discovered that genetic changes seen in ovarian cancers had evolved from cells lining the fallopian tube years earlier (maybe even several years prior). By looking at the genetic "signature" in cancer cells, they established their origin from the fallopian tube.

Based on this body of research, most

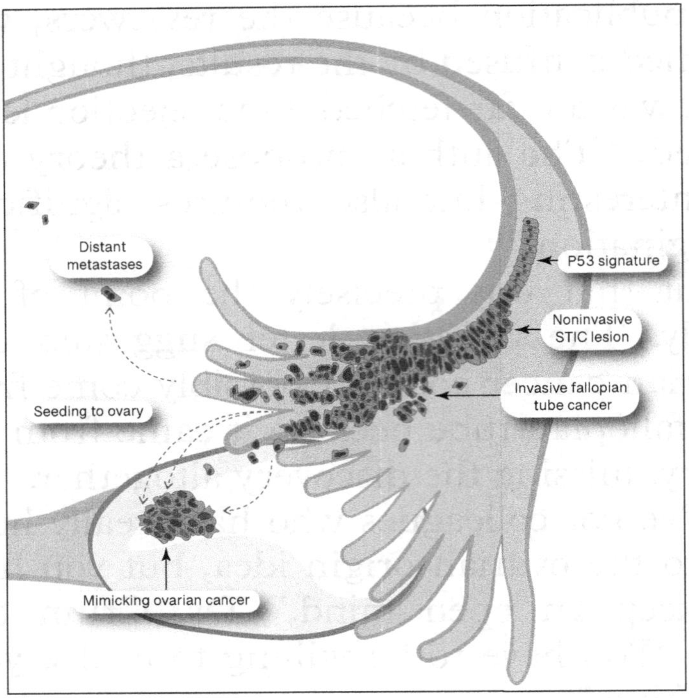

Newly recognized origin of ovarian cancer
(ILLUSTRATION BY CAROLYN HRUBAN)

gynecologists now recognize that the most common type of ovarian cancer arises from the inner lining of the fallopian tube. From there, the cells shower onto the ovary. It also explains why this cancer spreads in the free abdominal cavity quickly.

Over the past 60 to 70 years, doctors have removed millions of healthy ovaries from women worldwide in the name of preventing ovarian cancer. The discovery of the true origin of ovarian cancer had enormous implications for its prevention and treatment. In fact, it's turning the field upside down.

Save an Organ

Doctors previously assumed that ovaries have no function after a woman's childbearing years. They were wrong about that as well. It's well known that the ovaries produce high levels of hormones until menopause. But even after menopause, when hormone production drops precipitously, women still produce *lower* levels of hormones that can have some cardiovascular benefits and other health benefits. In other words, ovaries can still serve a purpose after menopause.

But this fact goes against historical dogma — dogma in line with the general underappreciation of health issues in women and consistent with medicine's traditional male-dominated mindset. I was reminded of the persistence of this mindset when a male physician with whom I was speaking about this discovery at a conference asked me, "Why is it a big deal for a woman to keep her ovaries after having children?"

In response, I asked him how we as men would feel if female surgeons removed men's testicles after we were finished having children.

He nodded slowly and winced. Now he could see it.

A good argument could be made that taking out healthy ovaries was the best recommendation based on the best available science available at the time. But here's what's hard to accept: Decades after the science was clear, surgeons are *still* taking out healthy ovaries in low-risk women.

How This Changed My Practice

I've walked over to the cancer center at Johns Hopkins thousands of times. But one day I had an extra pep in my step. I went to meet Dr. Velculescu, to talk to him about his 2017 study.

In his office, I asked him about his research. He explained that one of the reasons he had been willing to challenge the assumed origins of ovarian cancer was because modern medicine had been making no progress against this cruel disease. "Ovarian cancer treatments haven't changed much in many decades," he told me. "This may be, in part, because we have been studying the wrong tissue of origin for these cancers." Wow. It all made sense.

Discovering the tubal origin of the cancer was not just a theoretical breakthrough. It had huge real-world benefits. Doctors could now just remove the fallopian tubes and leave the ovaries in place, assuming the patient didn't have another reason to have them removed. Of course, this should only be considered when a woman is finished having children. We now know that routinely removing normal ovaries in low-risk women is overkill.

Based on this new information, all of our Johns Hopkins gynecology surgeons now generally offer most women the option to have their tubes removed when they have a hysterectomy, leaving the ovaries intact (if there are no other special circumstances). Similarly, women who come in and ask to have their tubes tied are now recommended to have them removed instead. (These women can still get pregnant via in vitro fertilization if they change their mind because the procedure spares the ovaries.) In fact, the American College of Obstetricians and Gynecologists has issued a new guideline recommending removal of the fallopian tube (sparing the ovary) for post-reproductive-age women having other gynecologic surgery.[7,8] That's because removing the fallopian tubes reduces their 1 in 78 chance of developing ovarian cancer in the future.

The fallopian tube is one of few anatomical structures that has no function or purpose other than for reproduction. That's why in my surgical practice, when I am discussing gallbladder removal or another abdominal procedure with a woman who's finished having kids, I now add a second conversation. I offer them the opportunity to talk to one of my gynecology colleagues about coming in during my procedure to remove their fallopian tubes. Ever since I learned of the new tubal origins research by Drs. Stone, Velculescu, and others, I continue to be amazed at how an additional 15-minute procedure can potentially save lives. To put it in context, removing the fallopian tubes is at least ten times more protective against cancer than a screening mammogram and colonoscopy *combined.*

Dr. Drapkin told me the discovery of ovarian cancer's origin in the fallopian tubes illustrates the importance of getting multiple perspectives. Most of his cancer research solicits input from scientists of a multitude of different backgrounds — physics, biochemistry, genetics, and other specialties — seeking fresh ideas and new approaches to crack the code on cancer. "Don't let yourself get boxed in," he told me. "If we all drink the same Kool-Aid, we're never going to discover anything new."

Dr. Drapkin is now studying the nerves

connected to tumors. He and his team have found that the activation of these nerves can contribute to tumor growth, suggesting a novel approach to tumor suppression.[9,10] Pretty cool.

The Opportunity

In parts of Canada and Germany, offering fallopian tube removal preemptively has already become standard of care for post-childbearing women having abdominal surgery. Starting in 2010, Canadian doctors adopted the new practice after Dr. Crum and the Dutch pathologists published their early findings. But U.S. adoption of this practice has lagged behind.

Canadian doctors are closely tracking their patient outcomes — and generating lessons for the world as a result. Last year, doctors at the University of British Columbia presented results of 80,000 women, 45% of whom had their tubes removed (leaving their ovaries intact) and 55% of whom were in a control group (having hysterectomy surgery that left their tubes and ovaries intact).[11] Of the women who'd had their tubes removed, only one developed a serous cancer, compared to 19 women in the group that had not had their tubes removed. In other words, removing the tubes resulted in a 93% reduction in serous cancer, the most common lethal type.

When I spoke with the study's lead author, Dr. Gillian Hanley, she told me that while serous ovarian cancers originate in the tubes, new research is revealing that two other subtypes of cancer may originate from the uterus (not the ovary). Removing the fallopian tubes likely cuts off the path by which these cancers spread.

There are other, less common (generally more benign) tumor types that can grow out of the ovary itself. For that reason, it's believed that removal of the fallopian tube (while sparing the ovaries) significantly reduces overall risks — although not entirely. Dr. Hanley says overall risk reduction for all tumor types is expected to be about 80%.[12,13]

Despite this benefit, many health care professionals are unaware of this new best practice. The American College of Obstetricians and Gynecologists states that removing the fallopian tubes "offers the opportunity to significantly decrease the risk of ovarian cancer." They also point out that leaving the ovaries in place enables women to benefit from the low levels of hormones that continue to come from the ovaries.

So let's do some math. In the U.S. about 400,000 women will have a hysterectomy each year and approximately 700,000 will have their tubes tied. Add to that a few million women who have abdominal surgery, like gallbladder or colon surgery, at an age after they're finished having children. All these operations offer the biggest opportunity we've ever had to lower ovarian cancer deaths.

Dr. Rebecca Stone told me about modeling data that suggested 2,000 lives a year could be saved by simply removing a woman's fallopian tubes (sparing the ovaries) at the time of hysterectomy, or in lieu of tying one's tubes. This would also save approximately half a billion dollars (ovarian cancer care costs an average of $1.5 million per patient), not to mention it would lighten the burden of chemotherapy and surgery. One University of Virginia study looking at the opportunity to remove the tubes during three common abdominal operations estimated that the approach could lower ovarian cancer rates by 28 to 38% on a national level.[14] Another study put the reduction estimate at 35 to 64%.[15]

What other new intervention in oncology slashes cancer rates by a third? In Canada, the gynecologists are now training general surgeons to safely remove the fallopian tubes when appropriate. (You would be surprised how many doctors confuse it with a nearby ligament called the round ligament of the uterus at quick glance.)

"I can't think of a time in medicine when we've had the opportunity to reduce the risk or even prevent a lethal cancer — a cancer that has no hope of effective screening on the horizon — by doing a simple surgery," Dr. Stone has said. "If you had the equivalent of this for pancreas cancer, it would be like a holy grail, yet the fact that salpingectomy [removal of fallopian tubes] has not been embraced by medicine in general says something," she commented. Some things in medicine are met with strong enthusiasm while other things encounter walls of disinterest. She and Dr. Joe Sakran are now leading collaborations in our hospital to bring this option to more women, starting with educating doctors and the general public.[16] Dr. Stone heads an international consortium of doctors to further study the issue and raise awareness.

The case to advance this message was bolstered in 2021 when a UK study reaffirmed that there is no effective screening test for ovarian cancer. The study of 200,000 women found that modern radiographic imaging and blood tests failed to identify women with early ovarian cancer.[17]

Couples Seeking Permanent Birth Control

My talks with several gynecologists suggested another implication of this new discovery. Historically, when a monogamous couple comes to the doctor seeking permanent birth control, the general recommendation has been that the male should have a vasectomy, assuming both are in good health. But a vasectomy does not reduce cancer risk. A fallopian tube removal does. So the recent discovery about the cancer-risk-reducing opportunity with fallopian tube removal tips the scale in favor of women having the procedure in lieu of men having a vasectomy. Of course, there are many other potential factors that could come into play in making this recommendation. But at a minimum, it alters the decision-making ledger.

Where Is This Going?

If you're a woman reading this chapter, you may be wondering whether you should have your fallopian tubes removed as a standalone procedure. In other words, if it's effective, why only offer it to women as an add-on to another operation?

This is a good question that the medical profession is not ready to answer. Leaders in this field are careful to say they do not recommend the operation as a stand-alone procedure just yet, even if it might be a powerful preventive measure. The hesitation may be more a function of the enormous societal implications of making such a sweeping recommendation.

Recommending that every woman in the world have an operation is a big deal. The health care system doesn't have the capacity, the quality control, or the definitive evidence to support such a massive public health recommendation — despite the fact that it's been a quarter century since the tubal origin of ovarian cancer was first suggested. You would think we would have larger population studies by now, but the stark reality is that things move slowly (too slowly). We will know more when we see the next wave of trial data from Canada.

Every medical intervention has risks. The question is: What are the trade-offs? A woman having the procedure will markedly reduce her 1.3% risk of ovarian cancer, but she will accept a roughly 0.01 to 0.001% risk of death or disability from the procedure itself (depending on the surgeon and other uncontrollable factors), and a roughly 1% risk of a minor surgical complication. Is that worth it? On a mass scale, no one is ready to say for certain until we have more data.

For starters, complication rates can vary by surgeon and if 1 in 100 surgeons has a very high complication rate, it could wipe out the entire community benefit of doing it as a stand-alone procedure.

There are other considerations. The risk of cancer varies in women, based on age and other factors. And the risk of an operation is different for each woman. The average age of women diagnosed with ovarian cancer is 63, suggesting that prevention after that age has a much lower yield. Also, surgery presents a higher risk for older women. By contrast, removing a 45-year-old woman's fallopian tubes would have a greater risk-reduction benefit and a lower risk of surgical complications. Identifying the sweet-spot age range of benefit-to-risk will help guide a broader recommendation.

Women at high risk for developing ovarian cancer may have a strong family history or a gene mutation. In some of these cases, a surgeon may recommend removing fallopian tubes *and* the ovaries. Taking out ovaries can be good medical care in certain circumstances. It depends on a woman's age, risk factors for developing ovarian cancer, hormone levels or hormone replacement therapy, and the potential concern of any abnormality seen on the ovary. Giving these women hormone replacement therapy after their ovaries are removed often helps them feel better and live longer.

As I spoke with gynecology oncology experts, it was clear that they grasped the magnitude of the potential broader recommendation for healthy women to have their tubes removed. Asking any healthy person, who has nothing wrong with them, to come into the hospital and have a minor procedure is a line in medicine that we rarely cross. We should only do it when there is a clear benefit that far outweighs the risks.

But putting aside all the logistical considerations, it does seem strange that this cancer-prevention procedure is highly recommended if you come in and ask to have your tubes tied, but not if you don't.

I will refrain from recommending that healthy women have the procedure after they are finished having kids. But if I were a woman contemplating permanent birth control, I would certainly carefully weigh the risks and benefits. We don't know the exact numbers yet, but at a distance, a risk of roughly 0.01 to 0.001% seems a lot more attractive than a risk of 1.3%. Other factors can also change over time. The rate of ovarian cancer is one of the few cancer rates that is rising. The number of ovarian cancer deaths has been projected to increase by approximately 50% over the next 20 years.[18,19]

After taking out millions of healthy ovaries for nearly a century in the name of cancer prevention, the medical profession's discovery that the most common form of ovarian cancer arises from the fallopian tubes has massive implications.

The Worst Name

Modern medicine is good at a lot of things, but naming things is not one of them. You have a "widowmaker," a certain nerve conduction pathway in the heart. You need a "fecal transplant." Or you have "triple negative" breast cancer, meaning each of three major hormone receptors is missing. These are just a few of the unfortunate descriptions we've cooked up for medical conditions and treatments. While such names may be helpful for medical professionals, they can confuse or distress patients.

When I heard that doctors recently coined the term "opportunistic salpingectomy" I once again smacked my forehead. Yes, that's the name for this new approach of removing the tubes while sparing the ovary. Salpingectomy means removal of the fallopian tubes. Fine. "Opportunistic" has a number of negative connotations. An opportunistic infection spreads in people whose immune defenses are down. The word also suggests taking advantage of a situation — an idea that may resonate negatively in poor and minority communities where a past generation of white male surgeons removed Black women's ovaries without their consent. As I asked people what they thought of the name, I discovered that doctors liked it and the public did not.

Step one in educating the public is to get a better name for the procedure — a name that appropriately describes it as a risk-reducing, ovary-sparing procedure. Hopefully, something will catch on to replace "opportunistic salpingectomy," which, to my dismay, increasingly dominates the research literature. You may wonder why I'm adamant about getting the name right. It should make more sense when you read the next page.

Moreover, perhaps we should also change the name of the cancer itself. For the majority of subtypes that originate in the fallopian tube, we might logically call them "fallopian tube cancer." That would be more accurate in most cases than "ovarian cancer."

Winning Back Trust

Medicaid does not allow doctors to remove the fallopian tubes without consent from the patient documented 30 days prior to the procedure. Why the emphasis on getting patient consent far in advance of the procedure? Unfortunately, there is a dark history of doctors removing ovaries and fallopian tubes without consent.

The eugenics movement in the United States led to some abhorrent practices in the late 19th and early 20th centuries. Eugenicists promoted breeding the most "desirable" type of children, and their practices included sterilizing men and women to prevent the transmission of "undesirable" traits, such as insubordination or alcoholism.[20] In 1907 Indiana became the first state to force or coerce sterilizations by policy based on eugenic principles. By 1931, 30 states had similar laws. Thousands of women each year had procedures to sterilize them, and most were poor and people of color. Eugenics subsided by the 1950s, but it continued under different names. It took until 1979 for regulations prohibiting sterilization under federally funded programs to take effect.[21] It's a shameful history, rooted in the paternalistic culture of medicine.

These shameful practices continued until much more recently in other countries. Between 1996 and 2000, Peru's government paid doctors and hospitals to perform forced-sterilization operations on an estimated 270,000 Indigenous women. That's right, this happened in the 1990s! Doctors tricked women into having surgery and removed their ovaries or tied their fallopian tubes without them knowing. Some were held down and forced to undergo the procedure. In other cases, women who went in for other routine procedures were sterilized as an add-on without their knowledge. As a result, a generation of young women were never able to conceive. This barbaric program was disguised as a public health program to address "population health." Peruvian doctors violated the sacred trust of the profession and used their authority to take advantage of women to participate in a medical genocide.[22,23]

Many of these women never had children, and many of the doctors who are alive today are still in practice. Despite having participated in the human rights violation, the doctors have not apologized, and no one has been punished. On the contrary, they were rewarded. Hospitals and doctors had been paid by the government based on the number of sterilization procedures they performed.

President Alberto Fujimori was president of Peru during this forced sterilization campaign, although he denied knowledge of the program. When his daughter Keiko Fujimori ran for president in 2016, it was a major issue for her campaign. Tens of thousands of women demonstrated in protest. She claims she was unaware of the sterilization campaign and believed in reparation payments for these women, but she failed to convince the people and lost the election. Her father, who was serving a 25-year prison term for human rights abuses, was released from prison on December 6, 2023, after the country's supreme court upheld a pardon he had received years prior.

It pains me to write this story as much as it may pain you to read it. We must never underestimate the potential for medical paternalism to escalate to crimes against humanity. Peru is an extremely poor country. At a minimum, doctors in Peru who were paid to participate in forced sterilization should be punished and pay the many women they mutilated. We as physicians must *always* abide by the principles of patient autonomy, transparency, and first, do not harm. We must also be wise in the way we communicate with the public, cognizant of the fact that many people have a reason or past family experience to be suspicious of medical experts.

There may also be less invasive ways in the future to remove or even ablate the fallopian tubes. Precision technology may also enable doctors to pinpoint the end of the tube closest to the ovary where cancer originates. There's one group at West Virginia University that has even removed fallopian tubes through the vagina.[24] That's right, no skin incision. Some believe this approach could reduce the reluctance for some women to have the procedure.

In this book, I do not give medical advice. But if my mother were younger and were having elective surgery on the abdomen with a good surgeon, I'd probably encourage her to ask about the procedure. Fallopian tube removal and sparing the ovary may represent a unique approach to reducing pain and premature death in the world.

When I think back over how far we've come in our approach to cancer, I'm proud of the medical profession. The creativity of the doctors that dare to think differently and discover new ways of thinking should be an inspiration to all scientists. I opened the chapter talking about Dr. B's powerlessness and frustration. Ovarian cancer is still an awful disease, but doctors no longer need to routinely remove healthy ovaries to combat it. We can be more precise. Over the coming years, it may become a more widely recommended add-on procedure. Until then, you may need to ask about it. And as more research data comes in, doctors should be ready to share it with the public, along with all their options, in real time.

It may be that a 15-minute procedure could dramatically reduce ovarian cancer deaths.

CHAPTER 9

Silicone Valley

Breast implants, autoimmune diseases, and the opioid crisis

Words are, of course,
the most powerful drug
used by mankind.
— Rudyard Kipling

Every now and then, I'll ask one of my surgical partners about one of our former residents. "Whatever happened to so-and-so? What are they up to these days?" Often the answer is that they're now in a leadership role at a top U.S. hospital or pioneering groundbreaking research.

One day when operating, I had a flashback to working with a former resident I'll call Joe. We all loved working with Joe because he had gifted hands and a genius for research. We felt he might someday cure cancer or do something big, given his work on cancer genetics while at Johns Hopkins. I reminisced with a colleague about how great it had been working with Joe.

"Whatever happened to Joe? What's he up to nowadays?" I asked.

My colleague responded, "He's very busy doing one thing — boob jobs in Miami."

"For real?" I looked at him in shock. The field of cancer had lost a great surgeon-scientist. We have trained so many talented surgeons who subsequently rush to the field of cosmetic surgery. In our lifetime, the demand for surgery to look better has soared. And for the last 50 years, the number one major plastic surgery requested by the public is breast augmentation — a procedure performed nearly a thousand times a day in the U.S.

Over a 30-year period, more than a million women chose to have a silicone breast implant operation.[1] About a fifth of them had the procedure to restore their figure after cancer surgery. Others simply wanted them for self-esteem, to look more attractive, particularly in certain parts of the U.S. We surgeons sometimes refer to the Miami–to–Palm Beach corridor as "Silicone Coast," and we call the Los Angeles–to–San Diego corridor "Silicone Valley."

Non-silicone-filled implants were tried, including those filled with saline, but women strongly preferred silicone implants because of their softness and natural look.

But then in 1992, the use of silicone implants came to a screeching halt. A national debate about the safety of the implant ignited. It was as religious as it was scientific and it raged for a decade, forever changing the field of medicine. A media grenade and government action created a pile-on effect that birthed the modern era of mass medical litigation. And out of the smoke emerged an opioid crisis that plagues the U.S. to this day.

This chapter of modern medicine began with a TV episode.

Connie Chung's Forest Fire

News anchor Connie Chung put silicone breast implants on center stage in America. Millions of Americans, mostly women, religiously watched her long-form exposés. She reported many milestone moments, but her December 10, 1990, broadcast on "breast implant illness," watched live by 13 million Americans,[2] would become her most popular.

Chung began the segment talking about breast implants, a potentially salacious topic that drives up ratings. "We've heard the rumors about which celebrities have them and which don't. But we don't know anything about the dangers."

Chung went on to profile multiple women with illnesses they claimed were due to their silicone implants. One woman, Janice, was introduced limping. She'd had the operation 11 years prior. Chung said, "Today, she can barely walk, she's plagued with illness." Janice explained, "I suffer constant pain, constant fatigue." She was taking expensive medications to deal with her debilitating symptoms. Watching the tape of the episode, I was personally curious if one of those medications was an opioid, potentially contributing to her disability.

Another woman, Judy, had had breast implants after a double mastectomy. Approximately a year later, she developed "flu-like" symptoms, joint pain, and difficulty going up and down stairs. A doctor told her she had silicone-associated disease. Chung asked a pathologist how silicone could make the immune system go "haywire." There wasn't any scientific study showing that silicone migration can cause those types of symptoms.

In the most frightening case Chung presented Sybil, who'd had five operations, some presumably involving placing and removing silicone implants. The program showed a picture of her disfigured chest, with Chung saying that the series of procedures had left her "mangled and infected." But it was unclear if her complications had anything to do with the silicone implant. To me, it appeared to be a case of botched surgery.

It didn't matter that there wasn't scientific evidence backing the claims made in the report. The one-sided presentation made it seem obvious that silicone implants were causing a host of health problems. And if it had happened to these victims, many viewers worried, then these same health problems might be brewing inside millions of other women who had silicone implants, even if they were not yet experiencing symptoms.

The company that made the silicone breast implant had paid CBS to run an ad, responding to the Chung report. It was set to run after a re-airing of the segment, and it gave a more balanced version of the story. But CBS canceled the ad just before the episode ran without providing an explanation.[3]

The controversy over silicone implants erupted a little before my time as a surgeon, so I reached out to some older surgeons who lived through it to get their first-hand account. Dr. Doug Wagner was a busy plastic surgeon in Akron, Ohio, at the time of the controversy. He was president of a plastic surgery society that invited me to speak at their annual conference. I got lunch with him so I could get his take.

Dr. Wagner described how the frenzy had led more women to suddenly complain of "breast implant illness," a poorly defined syndrome that included a vague constellation of symptoms such as malaise, fatigue, not sleeping well, hair loss, upset stomach, and brain fog. The more the illness became publicized, the more women identified with at least one symptom on the list. Women began asking to have their silicone implants removed. They would then tell their friends who would sometimes do the same, spreading the practice even further.

"A lot of women got their silicone implants exchanged for saline implants," Dr. Wagner told me. "The irony is that silicone implants have fewer leaks than saline implants."

Dr. Wagner recalled one woman who had gone to him during the media buzz, asking him to remove her silicone implants. She said she had suffered from "breast implant illness" for the past year. Dr. Wagner pointed out that she'd had the implants for 20 years.

"Why didn't she have it the first 19 years?" he said. It seemed to him that women had begun attributing normal changes of aging to this novel idea of a disease.

"It's unclear if breast implant illness was a

real disease," Dr. Wagner explained. "Lawyers made it one because lawsuits against the manufacturer resulted in a requirement to warn patients about 'breast implant illness' before they had the procedure." This warning, in turn, gave the disease more legitimacy.

The warning became part of the informed consent and thus a part of the conversation about implant risks. It was a disease largely egged on by lawyers and magnified by doctors being forced to warn people about it. It took on a life of its own. As talk of "breast implant illness" increased, it spread like a virus. More and more women began to attribute any medical ailment to it. In any group of a million-plus women, approximately 40,000 to 50,000 women will develop connective tissue diseases *normally,* irrespective of having a silicone implant. But now with the buzz going around, those with an implant who developed a connective tissue disease, chronic fatigue syndrome, or any of a host of health issues (as many people normally do) believed it had been *caused* by the dangerous implants. According to Dr. Wagner, it was essentially a manufactured epidemic, a crisis that continues to this day, fueled by social media.

Connie Chung had started a forest fire.

Enter Dr. Kessler

The Connie Chung interview created a national health emergency. Days after the story, Congress held hearings on silicone breast implants. The only three scientific experts who testified at the hearing were paid expert witnesses for plaintiffs suing the silicone implant manufacturer.[4,5] Congressman Ted Weiss from New York wrote in a letter to FDA commissioner Dr. David Kessler, "the cancer risks [of silicone implants] . . . may be more than 100 times the levels reported by the FDA." Advocacy groups also weighed in against the implants.[6]

Thirteen months after Chung's episode, the FDA made a big move. Dr. Kessler, a former pediatrics resident from Johns Hopkins, announced a temporary moratorium, and then a ban, on silicone implants. "The FDA cannot assure the safety of these devices at this time," Kessler declared at a press conference in January 1992. "We still do not know how often the implants leak, and when they do; we do not know exactly what materials get into the body."[7] He also warned, "We still do not know whether the implants can increase a woman's risk of developing cancer. And we still do not know enough about the relationship between these devices and autoimmune and connective tissue diseases." These were strong warnings coming from the nation's top regulator of medical devices. The FDA concern that silicone implants could trigger an autoimmune disease came from a medical report of just three women.[8]

Oddly, silicone breast implants were still allowed to be used but only for reconstructive cancer surgery if the patient was registered in a clinical trial. Also, Kessler allowed *saline* implants to remain on the market.

Some of Kessler's opposition seemed to be based on a negative opinion of breast augmentation when done strictly for cosmetic purposes. "It makes little sense for the FDA to consider breast augmentation of equivalent importance with an accepted component of cancer therapy," he later wrote in the *New England Journal*.[9]

Kessler also warned in the same article that even a woman with no symptoms could have a "silent rupture,"[10] instilling even more anxiety in the million-plus women with the implant. He told all women with the implant to have periodic checkups for problems such as implant rupture.

Now women had two people making them worried sick: Connie Chung and the nation's top medical regulator. Over the subsequent years, the fears snowballed into an avalanche.

The media gave these worries a megaphone. The *Los Angeles Times* reported that "silicone implants may cause serious health problems in women — and, perhaps, even in some of their children."[11] Many other media outlets reported the same fears, blindly parroting the safety concerns coming from the government.

The media and the government, almost in lockstep, ignited a nationwide frenzy. Thousands of women lined up to have their silicone breast implants surgically removed. One retired Johns Hopkins plastic surgeon told me some younger women with naturally small breasts had struggled emotionally with the loss of their breast implants in the same way women struggle after having a bilateral mastectomy. "Marty, you can't imagine what it did to their self-esteem," he told me.

Demand for breast implant removal was so high that the Government Accountability Office wrote a letter to Congress urging Medicaid and other federally funded insurance programs to cover the procedures.[12] Some women swapped their silicone implants for saline implants. Dr. Kessler suggested that only a small number of women *preferred* silicone over saline, even though women have always preferred the look and feel of silicone.[13]

Doctors Push Back

Dr. Kessler was widely respected. But quickly, another prominent American physician became vocal on the issue. Dr. Marcia Angell, who would later become the editor in chief of the *New England Journal,* took issue with Dr. Kessler's ominous warnings and regulatory actions. She criticized the FDA's ban, arguing that the implants had been in use for 30 years with minimal side effects and widespread satisfaction.[14] She also pointed out that Kessler's ban had "given rise to great fears among the one million women living with implants" that were out of proportion with the risks. She suggested that Kessler, with his apparent bias against cosmetic implants, was "holding the implant to an impossibly high standard: since there was no benefit, there should be no risks."

Prominent leaders of the American Society of Plastic Surgeons agreed. They took issue with Kessler's pronouncements, arguing there was insufficient data to pull them off the open market.

Doctors pointed to the fact that the existing data and the 30-year experience of the implant in over a million women suggested they were safe. They acknowledged that an earlier version of the implant had had a slightly higher leak rate, but the more durable version being used at the time had a strong safety profile. Some doctors who were perplexed by the ban assumed the FDA must have had non-public data because it's the only way Kessler's extreme action made sense.

Dr. Norman Cole, who served as president of the American Society of Plastic Surgeons at the time, told the *New York Times,* "To us [this] is very disturbing, and sends a very negative message to patients that there is something wrong with these implants . . . If there has been new and significant scientific data, we want to know what it is. We don't have it."

Dr. Mitchell Karlan, a prominent California physician, objected to Kessler's decision, telling reporters, "There will be absolute hysteria among women . . . We already have the data, the experience of physicians."

After Dr. Kessler banned silicone implants for cosmetic purposes, he continued to make his case. The following year, Kessler wrote another article defending his position, this time in the *Journal of the American Medical Association,* as the debate raged for years.[15]

The silicone breast implant issue seemed to occupy an inordinate amount of regulatory focus during Dr. Kessler's term at the FDA. In contrast, almost no attention was paid to MS Contin, a long-acting opioid whose sales had begun to increase. The agency had deemed MS Contin safe and effective just four years prior to Kessler's silicone implant ban and had approved it for widespread use. While Kessler demanded long-term studies on silicone breast implants, no such demand was made of opioid products.

One year into Kessler's ban on silicone implants, his agency began its evaluation of Purdue Pharma's application for OxyContin. The next year, the agency approved the highly addictive drug with the belief that it "would result in *less* abuse potential" according to the agency.[16] The approval was based on a 14-day clinical trial in people with osteoarthritis. No effort was made by the FDA to monitor the drug for complications like dependency.

The FDA's website describes its approval in December 1995 in this way: "FDA believed the controlled-release formulation of OxyContin would result in *less* abuse potential."[17] But this opinion was not based on any valid data. It was simply

Purdue Pharma's claim, and Kessler's FDA bought it.

The FDA's Dr. Janet Woodcock oversaw the division that approved OxyContin. Perdue Pharma promised that it would do another study and submit the results to the FDA but it never did.[18] For the next 23 years, Dr. Woodcock let them off the hook for breaking their promise.

Evidence that OxyContin was safe and effective in treating chronic pain was nonexistent, and still is. In short, OxyContin's approved label to treat patients for chronic pain was scientifically flawed.

Ironically, some women who had surgery to remove their silicone breast implants were prescribed excessive doses of opioids. We all did it. It was the groupthink that was beaten into me as a surgical resident. The dogma was supported by a frequently cited 1980 letter in the *New England Journal* declaring that "addiction was rare."[19] It's likely that some women died not from the silicone but from the opioids they were given for their alleged breast implant illness.

The debate about silicone implants continued for years but there was little debate about opioids. Some doctors were concerned that opioids could be addictive, but they were seen as antiestablishment. The

American Pain Society and other groups repeated the dogma. Purdue Pharma sales reps approached doctors who were skeptical that OxyContin was less addictive, but the reps were often able to convince the doctors of the drug's benefits after citing the FDA's approved label. No long-term studies of opioid dependence were required by Kessler or the FDA throughout his term, which lasted until 1997 — the longest term of any FDA commissioner in the last half century.

Ironically, OxyContin was approved by the FDA for chronic use based on a 14-day clinical trial, as silicone breast implants were effectively kept off the market for not showing the FDA long-term outcome data.

It would not be until 2017 that the medical field would be humbled by a study that was embarrassingly simple. Researchers at the University of Michigan looking at pharmacy fill records found that 1 in 16 patients who were given opioids after surgery were still taking opioids three to six months later.[20] Some doctors had long known that opioids were addictive,[21] but this Michigan study detailed how minor surgical procedures could spark the addiction. It was a wake-up call. The study was also so simple to conduct and so revealing, that it's maddening to think it could have been easily done prior to the opioid epidemic.

Lawyers Cashing In

The silicone implant controversy birthed a new phenomenon in America: mass medical tort (litigation). Lawyers seized on the chaos. They affirmed the beliefs of women fixated on their silicone implant as the cause of their life's woes. They built upon a precedent case from 1984 in which a court ordered the manufacturer Dow Corning to pay $1.5 million in punitive damages after Maria Stern claimed the silicone implant had caused her autoimmune disease.

The Stern case went largely unnoticed until Connie Chung broadcast her expose.[22] Then came a wave of lawsuits against the manufacturer that would consume the company for more than a decade.

The FDA's ban gave the trial lawyers additional ammo.

Two years into Kessler's ban, a Houston jury awarded $27.9 million to three women who claimed they suffered from atypical lupus, neurological impairment, and a "silicone induced" autoimmune problem. By the end of that year, more than 19,000 lawsuits had been filed against the maker of the silicone implant.

By 1995, 440,000 women had registered in

a global settlement. Dow Corning eventually agreed to pay $3.2 billion to settle claims.[23] It was the largest medical injury settlement ever at the time.

Plaintiff's attorneys Stanley Chesley and John O'Quinn had built mass empires from the litigation. They would become known as pioneers of mass medical tort.

"Once the trial lawyers got involved, it got a life of its own," Dr. Bill Crawley, a plastic surgeon affiliated with Johns Hopkins who practiced at the time, told me.

Despite all the buzz, evidence was never presented that silicone breast implants caused any woman to suffer lupus, cancer, or another condition.

A Manufactured Epidemic

The size of the opioid crisis was downplayed as the size of the breast implant illness epidemic was overplayed. But soon, studies began to discredit claims that silicone implants cause autoimmune and other diseases. In 1994, the Mayo Clinic published a large *New England Journal* study concluding, "We found no association between breast implants and the connective-tissue diseases and other disorders that were studied."[24] The next year, the American College of Rheumatology stated it did not see compelling evidence of any cause-and-effect relationship between silicone breast implants and connective tissue disease. The American College of Neurology issued a similar statement. The increased risk of breast cancer was also disproven in several studies. And in a surprise twist, a review published in the *Journal of the National Cancer Institute* found that existing studies "actually suggest that breast cancer risk might be reduced among women with implants."[25]

The data were clear. They had affirmed what surgeons had been saying for years: Silicone implants had a low risk of "local" complications and did not cause autoimmune disease, cancer, or other chronic conditions.

Four years into Kessler's ban, Dr. Marcia Angell, who had sparred with Kessler in the *New England Journal,* published the book *Science on Trial: The Clash of Medical Evidence and the Law in the Breast Implant Case*. The book raised awareness of the lack of scientific merit behind the FDA's ban, while body-slamming the courts for making judgments with no scientific backing.

"There is clearly a disparity between the little that has been demonstrated about the risks and the abundance of anecdotes now being related in the media and the courts," Angell wrote.

Angell also criticized the FDA for fear-mongering and pointed out the potential sexism in Kessler's decision. She explained that one reason for the double standard was that the benefits of silicone implants were not as tangible as they would be for a typical medication the FDA oversaw. A medication will often improve a patient's symptoms, cure or lessen their disease, or make other recordable changes. Implants, however, were often used to boost self-esteem and self-confidence, especially in women who'd had to receive a mastectomy due to cancer or another ailment, Angell argued.

Angell and others pointed out that substances like alcohol and tobacco — which kill more than a hundred thousand Americans each year — remain widely available, while devices used to improve a woman's mental health were stripped away with little evidence. Supporters of Kessler argued that he had taken on the tobacco industry more forcefully than anyone ever has (Kessler is also credited with approving HIV medications relatively quickly). Dr. Angell went on to be a leading patient advocate and critic of FDA policy. Her advocacy efforts challenging the FDA's silicone ban earned her the distinction of being named one of *Time* magazine's 25 most influential Americans in 2001.[26]

Dr. William Dupont of Vanderbilt University also criticized Kessler's war on silicone implants. He warned that Kessler's decision would "have a profound impact on our society if it [were to be] applied consistently to other devices." He pointed out that contact lenses are cosmetic and can have severe adverse effects. "Will the FDA continue to tolerate this practice?" he asked. Kessler responded to Dupont, saying the comparison between the implants and contact lenses was unfair and that there was research at the time showing contacts were safe and effective.[27]

I reached out to Dr. Kessler and asked him what his thoughts were on the saga. Ahead of our conversation, he emailed me a 2023 article suggesting that a rare type of lymphoma has been implicated with a textured version of the silicone implant.[28] He told me he stands by his decision, though it had been a difficult one, and pointed out that the implant manufacturers had had ample time to submit safety data before the ban but that they had failed to do so. He also told me that the ban was designed to get more information and was consistent with the law.

The Final Word

By 1996, a growing number of silicone implant lawsuits had made their way to federal court. It was a culmination point in the national battle over silicone implants. Judge Sam C. Pointer oversaw the cases and decided to get to the bottom of the science. He appointed a national science panel to review the best available medical studies and issue a report. After two years, the panel concluded that scientific evidence had failed to show that silicone breast implants cause disease. The judge's creation of a scientific panel ushered in a new era of scientific standards to the courtroom, now termed the Daubert standard, which has since improved the quality of expert witness testimony.[29]

The next year, 1999, the Institute of Medicine (later re-named the National Academy of Medicine) issued a 400-page report written by 13 independent scientists.[30] The report concluded that while silicone implants can cause some minor problems like hardening of the breast or scar tissue, they do not cause any major diseases, including autoimmune disease.

The billion-dollar war on silicone was now over.

Where We Are Today

In 1998, Dr. Kessler admitted to the *New York Times* that "There's no evidence that [silicone breast implants] cause systemic disease."[31] But by that time, the manufacturer Dow Corning had already filed for Chapter 11 bankruptcy.

After Kessler's ban, no other company would risk bringing another silicone breast implant to market. But eventually one company dared to make the implant again. In 2006, the FDA lifted its 14-year ban and issued its first approval of a silicone implant. Again, the silicone implant emerged to be the preferred implant of choice by women because of its softness and natural feel. Of note, the FDA at the time did not allow the implant to be used for augmentation in women under age 22. The agency would soon become known for vindictive actions against companies, punishing company's actions around one of their products by pulling another one of their product's off the market. In 2010, three years after Kessler's departure, the FDA began to spy on its own scientists who expressed safety concerns about device approvals; four whistleblowers were fired.[32] The agency accessed their private emails using spyware that took screenshots of their laptops every five seconds.

Stanley Chesley, one of the plaintiff's attorneys in the breast implant cases, became known as "the master of disaster" for representing victims of fires, plane crashes, and alleged medical malfeasance. His career ended in disgrace after he was disbarred for helping attorneys get exorbitant fees, cheating clients, and then lying about it in a coverup.[33]

John O'Quinn, another of the plaintiff's attorneys who's been referred to as the "king of torts," went on to own 200 automobiles housed in seven warehouses.[34] He was later ordered to repay $41 million that he had overcharged his breast implant clients.[35] He died in a 2009 automobile accident. In a dark irony, he was not wearing a seat belt.[36]

Since the approval of OxyContin by Kessler's FDA, the opioid epidemic is believed to have killed more than 1 million Americans. Dr. Janet Woodcock, who led the FDA division that approved OxyContin for chronic pain (despite zero data that it worked for chronic pain) was subsequently promoted to lead the agency from 2021 to 2022 as FDA acting commissioner. Prior to her taking the top job, a coalition of 28 public health groups and opioid crisis organizations sent a letter to the White House asking that she *not* lead the agency. The letter stated that "Dr. Woodcock presided over one of the worst regulatory agency failures in U.S. history."[37]

Dr. Kessler went on to become the dean

of Yale School of Medicine after he left the FDA. Five years later he became the dean of the medical school at the University of California San Francisco. In 2021, the White House named Dr. Kessler to be chief science adviser for the Covid response, a position he held until 2023.

The silicone breast implant war was costly, with much collateral damage. Medical journals became forums for the time-consuming debate, women experienced information whiplash and had countless operations as a result, and America's courts became flooded with litigation costing billions.

Today, 3% of U.S. women have breast implants, and silicone is once again the standard of care for breast implant surgery.

CHAPTER 10

A Comedy of Errors

A short history of medical groupthink

The good thing about science is that it's true whether or not you believe in it.

— Neil deGrasse Tyson

In my medical training, I was required to memorize how to do a number of complex operations to treat stomach ulcers. Some seemed barbaric. One involved cutting the body's longest two-way nerve, the vagus nerve, which connects the gut with the brain, and rerouting the patient's intestines. Ulcers were a common reason people landed in the hospital in those days. When patients asked what caused their ulcers, doctors responded with one word: "Stress."

The right answer would have been "We don't know."

In the early 1980s, Dr. Barry Marshall, a researcher in Australia, was studying the cause of ulcer disease. He was intrigued by a nonconventional idea — one that had been suggested in studies published over the previous hundred years. The studies speculated that ulcers were caused not by stress, but by a spiral bacteria. He read about a Greek physician named Dr. John Lykoudis who had success treating 10,000 ulcer patients with antibiotics in the 1960s only to have his medical license revoked because the treatment departed from accepted medical practice.[1]

The more Dr. Marshall learned, the more emboldened he became to challenge establishment thinking. He wanted to test the hypothesis that ulcers were caused by the bacteria and that they could be treated with a short course of antibiotics. But he faced powerful opposition. He tried several times to voice his perspective and got laughed out of the room.

So Dr. Marshall pursued his hypothesis on his own. He did a formal study on a series of ulcer patients. He even performed an experiment on himself! He drank the bacteria to give himself the disease and then had his stomach biopsied to prove the cause and effect. Then he cured himself with a short course of antibiotics. He did many other experiments that worked. He demonstrated that stomach ulcers were caused by one specific bacteria that he isolated:

Helicobacter pylori. It was one of the greatest breakthroughs in medicine. Instead of requiring major surgery, stomach ulcers could be cured with an antibiotic.

Dr. Marshall and his colleague, Dr. Robin Warren, submitted their bombshell findings for consideration at a medical conference, but they got this response:

> 17th March, 1983
>
> Dear Dr. Marshall,
>
> I regret that your research paper was not accepted for presentation . . .
>
> The number of abstracts we receive continues to increase and ***for this meeting 67 were submitted and we could only accept 56.***

Their discovery didn't even make the top 56! I wonder what the other ten rejected abstracts were about.

It would take tireless efforts by Drs. Marshall and Warren to get their cure in front of the medical community. By the early 1990s, nearly every doctor finally got on board because the data were so undeniable. Many lives were saved because of the courage and persistence of these two men. Their discovery is now heralded as one of the great breakthroughs in medicine. In 2005, they were awarded the Nobel Prize.

Groupthink is as old as the medical profession. It's part of the human condition. As I researched groupthink in medicine, I found no shortage of groundbreaking innovators throughout history who were sidelined for challenging conventional thinking. I read about dozens of groundbreaking scientists from centuries ago, all the way up to the doctor who invented the mRNA vaccine.

I gathered my notes and walked over to the History of Medicine department at Johns Hopkins, in the historic Welch Library. There I met with amazing scholars like Drs. Jeremy Greene and Mary Fissell, who regaled me with colorful stories and fascinating insights. We shared our astonishment as we noted the same patterns of medical elites ruling by edict and kneecapping the brave souls who challenged their dogma.

Starting with an account from medieval times and concluding with the modern-day development of mRNA vaccines, the stories that follow highlight a similar theme: The majority's urge to resist new ideas is powerful. Sometimes the resistance is so tragic it's funny — a comedy of errors. Dr. Festinger's concept of cognitive dissonance is on display throughout.

An Early Victim of Cancel Culture: Dr. Michael Servetus

In the Middle Ages, doctors believed the body turned food into blood, and blood just sat in the body stagnant. (I still think that's true of some of my early morning students sleeping in the front row.) Blood doesn't circulate, they believed. It would only be replaced by eating more food that then converted to blood. The heart — the pounding thing everyone could feel in their chests — was thought to be a source of heat.

But then in the 16th century, Spanish theologian Michael Servetus dared to postulate otherwise. Servetus wasn't shy of controversy. In a book called *The Restoration of Christianity,* he criticized the church. But what changed our understanding of the body was the bizarre addendum to his theological treatise in which he provided an accurate description of the body's circulatory system. I guess he tried to publish his theory anywhere he could.

It was a "good-news-bad-news" situation for Servetus.

The good news? His circulation theory turned out to be correct.

The bad news: His theological beliefs got him in trouble. John Calvin had him arrested for heresy and he was burned at the stake. Publish or perish, they say. Sadly for Servetus, it turned out to be both.

The "Crack-Brained" Genius: Dr. William Harvey

Dr. William Harvey was born 25 years after Servetus's execution. Since Servetus had been regarded as a heretical nut job, few took his circulation theory seriously. But Dr. Harvey didn't write him off. He objectively considered the circulation theory. Seeing what had become of poor Servetus, Dr. Harvey used a more data-driven approach.

Dr. Harvey was a British prodigy. At 16, he was awarded a scholarship to study medicine at Cambridge University, where he focused on Aristotle.[2] He also learned under a famous anatomist in Italy and became a rising figure among doctors in Europe.[3] Before the age of 30, Harvey was accepted into the Royal College of Physicians. Years later, he became a physician for King James I and then King Charles I. It sounds cool but trust me, VIP patients can be a pain in the butt.

Dr. Harvey conducted autopsies on animals and humans to learn more about the heart and circulatory system. In 1628, at age 50, Harvey published the culmination of his life's work.[4] He argued that the heart pumped a significant volume of blood with each contraction — too much blood for the body's tissue to absorb. The blood had to go somewhere! He theorized that it moved through the body and returned to the heart in a circle-like pattern, with the heart serving as the engine. He published mathematical calculations to show how it worked.

Naturally, Dr. Harvey got criticized for getting it exactly right. Many found his findings to be ludicrous. He said at the time that his practice took a big hit (in his words it "fell mightily") and that physicians were against his opinion.[5] Even worse, he was called "crack-brained," a term I gather, despite my ignorance of medieval vernacular, is not exactly a compliment.

Some historians have called Dr. Harvey's description of the circulatory system the greatest medical discovery of all time.[6]

And even better, he didn't get burned at the stake.

Eat Lemons: Dr. James Lind's Clinical Trial

Flying isn't exactly fun nowadays, especially when the pilot gets on the loudspeaker and interrupts a strategic catnap. Even more tragic, the announcement is just to inform you that the plane has reached an altitude of 31,000 feet. I don't care if you skim the trees, just get us there, I sometimes want to respond. But when I find myself irritated on a plane and then pushed over the edge by a hyperenthusiastic credit card offer announcement, it helps to pause and get a little historical perspective. For centuries, crossing the Atlantic by ship was rougher. Sometimes crews didn't even know where they would land. If you think a little turbulence is scary, consider storms with 20-foot waves, pirates, mutiny, or just getting lost at sea. Oh, and rats. There were always rats. I know the snacks on planes are a little stale, but let's be real. We'd rather dart across the Atlantic in six hours, watching movies in a climate-controlled cabin, than take our chances on the open seas.

But here's something surprising: The biggest peril of the sea wasn't squalls or pirates or shipwrecks. It was a different threat that killed millions: a lack of vitamin C.

Scurvy, a painful disease that erupts when a person lacks vitamin C, killed about two million sailors from Columbus's voyage in 1492 until the 1800s. Ships would sometimes lose half their men to the scourge, which was a mystery at the time.

The descriptions of scurvy sound like something from a horror movie. Naval crews got particularly hammered by it. Admiral

George Anson, a Royal Navy officer in the early 1700s, described the illness as a "luxuriancy of funguous flesh . . . [and] putrid gums."[7] He was probably referring to the bleeding gums and skin lesions associated with the disease. On one voyage, he lost 1,300 of his 2,000 men to scurvy.

Not exactly the same as picking up the sniffles on a domestic flight.

The diary of one English seaman who had scurvy and recovered, reported by the Science History Institute,[8] reads like a scene from *The Walking Dead:*

> It rotted all my gums, which gave out a black and putrid blood. My thighs and lower legs were black and gangrenous, and I was forced to use my knife each day to cut into the flesh in order to release this black and foul blood. I also used my knife on my gums, which were livid and growing over my teeth . . . When I had cut away this dead flesh and caused much black blood to flow, I rinsed my mouth and teeth with my urine, rubbing them very hard . . . And the unfortunate thing was that I could not eat, desiring more to swallow than to chew . . . Many of our people died of it every day, and we saw bodies thrown into the sea constantly, three or four at a time.

People who sailed to the Americas to flee the tyranny of monarchies had to weigh the risk of scurvy (maybe living under the tyranny of a king suddenly didn't seem that bad).

The world was dumbfounded by the disease, and it limited world trade, exploration (aka imperialism), and even the slave trade.[9] No doctor could figure out why a person would develop these horrendous and bizarre symptoms when out at sea. Some blamed the ocean air or the lack of exercise while at sea. There were competing theories about how to treat the condition, whether to drink cider, vinegar, or even seawater. Yuck.

Then along came Dr. James Lind, a curious man, who had a knack for the scientific method.[10] He joined the Royal Navy in 1738 as a "surgeon's mate" — effectively a member of the crew who was also medically trained and would work alongside the ship's chief surgeon.[11] By the way, "chief surgeon" sounds impressive, but they mostly did amputations and tooth extractions.

Dr. Lind had witnessed many seamen killed by scurvy and had heard rumors about possible treatments.[12] He decided to perform a controlled experiment, a clinical trial in 1747. While sailing on a ship named the *Salisbury,* he gathered 12 sailors with scurvy. He split them into pairs, and each of the six groups was treated with a different remedy for 14 days. Here are the six arms to his clinical trial:

1. Drinking 1.1 liters of cider (*doesn't sound too bad*)
2. Drinking a mixture of alcohol and sulfuric acid (*the acid is a tangy chaser*)
3. Taking a swig of vinegar before each of three meals (*sounds like a recipe for belching*)
4. Drinking a half-pint of seawater (*disgusting*)
5. Applying a medicinal paste of garlic, mustard seed, and dried radish seed (*sounds irresistible*)
6. Eating two oranges and one lemon every day (*seems out of left field*)

It's like the clinical trial was designed by Dr. Frankenstein.

Due to a lack of supplies, the orange and lemon group could only participate in the experiment for six of the 14 days. But luckily, six days was enough. In the book in which he later published his results, Dr. Lind wrote: "The most sudden and visible good effects were perceived from the use of oranges and lemons."

The book, titled *Treatise of the Scurvy,* was published in 1753, but sadly it was largely ignored. As a result, the cure to a global epidemic was rarely used. Some historians speculate that Dr. Lind was not vocal enough about his findings. It took more than 40 years after his first publication for the Royal Navy to start stocking lemon juice on its ships.

LISTEN TO THE FARMERS: DR. EDWARD JENNER

In the 18th century, an estimated 400,000 Europeans died from smallpox.[13]

Smallpox was much deadlier than Covid-19. The fatality rate of Covid over its first three years was approximately 0.1%. For smallpox it was 20 to 50%. Smallpox survivors sometimes lived with debilitating conditions, such as blindness. It was brutal. Worldwide, smallpox fostered imperialism as it decimated susceptible populations, such as Native Americans who acquired the disease from European settlers with higher levels of immunity.[14]

European health officials scratched their heads to figure out how to stop the spread, but farmers from the countryside had an idea. Farmers noticed that people infected with cowpox, a far milder disease, did not get smallpox. In particular, milkmaids, nearly all of whom had cowpox infection from working with cows, were renown for not getting smallpox. Based on their observations, the farmers suggested that cowpox infection provided subsequent "cross immunity" to smallpox.[15]

Did the sophisticated doctors listen to the "uneducated" farmers? No, they didn't. The elitist doctors laughed at the farmers, thinking they were ignorant.

But Dr. Edward Jenner, who grew up in the countryside, took their claim seriously. Rather than mocking them, he considered the idea with an open mind, and studied it. Over the course of 20 years, Jenner collected information on cowpox, smallpox, and how people could develop cross immunity.

In 1796, Dr. Jenner obtained live cowpox particles by scraping the cowpox blister of an infected milkmaid named Sarah Nelmes. He then scratched the arm of an 8-year-old son of his gardener, and rubbed it with the skin particles from Sarah Nelmes's cowpox blister. The boy became sick with the mild cowpox infection. Then, weeks later, after he recovered, Dr. Jenner exposed the young boy to cowpox again (what we refer to in medicine as a "challenge trial"). This time, the boy did not develop any symptoms, suggesting that the first exposure had provided immunity.

Dr. Jenner had just performed the first-ever vaccination.[16]

Dr. Jenner also observed that his cowpox particles also provided immunity against the dreaded smallpox.

The doctor reported his findings to the Royal Society, an elite institution for science and medicine in the UK. He had been admitted to the society nearly a decade earlier for controversial research on how the cuckoo bird reproduced — research initially ridiculed before being accepted as fact decades later.[17] That experience may have emboldened Dr. Jenner with the courage he needed to create the world's first vaccine and begin the centuries-long effort that would ultimately result in smallpox eradication.

The Royal Society has a rich tradition of being objective and open-minded to new ideas, but the people in power at the time rejected Dr. Jenner's research and warned that "he had better not promulgate such a wild idea if he valued his reputation."

Dr. Jenner was undeterred. He published a book summarizing the more than two decades of research he had performed on vaccinating people.[18] He told the story of 23 people who had been exposed to cowpox, and detailed how they went on to become immune to cowpox and smallpox. He described the cure to one of the greatest global pandemics in history, yet the Royal Society and other medical leaders rejected him as outlandish.

Still undeterred, Dr. Jenner traveled to London, hoping to perform larger human trials to further prove his vaccine theory correct. He coined the term "vaccine," a derivative of the Latin word *vacca,* for "cow." (I took four years of Latin because people said it would help in medical school. It did not, so I'm mentioning the Latin root here as "effort justification.") Dr. Jenner had trouble getting people to take his vaccine, at one point going three months without a single volunteer.

But gradually his patient outcomes spoke for themselves.

Dr. Jenner sent his vaccine samples to other trusted physicians. Benjamin Waterhouse, a physician and co-founder of Harvard Medical School, got Jenner's samples and inoculated his wife and children. Dr. Jenner happened to know President Johns Adams and asked him to consider a mass vaccination program.[19] But for unknown reasons, Adams did not respond to his request. At the same time, the world's first anti-vaxxers began to emerge, among them skeptical medical elites.

Dr. Waterhouse then pleaded his case to Vice President Thomas Jefferson. Jefferson endorsed the vaccine, writing, "Every friend of humanity must look with pleasure on this discovery."

As president, Jefferson eventually created the National Vaccine Institute, setting the stage for the mass administration of Jenner's smallpox vaccine. By the early 1900s, the disease was all but defeated in the United States and Europe.

By 1980, the WHO declared smallpox to be eradicated.[20] To this day, Dr. Jenner is considered the father of immunology. Researchers later built upon his findings to control measles, bubonic plague, and other infectious diseases. This unlikely discovery had been a direct result of Dr. Jenner's humility to listen to farmers. They were not "educated," but they were right.

The Tale of Two Clinics: Dr. Ignaz Semmelweis

In 1846, a Hungarian doctor, Ignaz Semmelweis, was working as a chief resident at the Vienna General Hospital.[21] The hospital had two nearby obstetrical clinics that provided free care to pregnant women, if they agreed to be examined by medical students as part of their training.[22] The two clinics served the same local population and took turns admitting patients on alternate days. Surprisingly, the first clinic had a bad reputation because about 10% of women treated there died of "childbed fever" — an infection of the woman's reproductive tract — but the second clinic had a mortality rate of less than 4%.

Women knew the reputation of the first clinic and feared it. Some were so afraid they elected to give birth outside on the street instead of in the ward. Even more strange, the women who gave birth on the street had a lower mortality rate than the women who gave birth in the more dangerous clinic.

Semmelweis had been studying the cause of the higher death rate, so his ears perked up when a friend of his suffered a tragic death.[23] His friend had been performing an autopsy when he accidentally was poked with a knife, which led to a fatal infection — the same infection that had been killing many pregnant women in the clinic.

Semmelweis made an important connection. His friend had died after working on a cadaver. Women from the more dangerous clinic had been examined by doctors who had also been working on cadavers, and the doctors did not wash their hands after working on the cadavers and before examining the patients. In contrast, the clinic with the lower mortality rate did not have doctors examining both dead bodies and young mothers.

Scientists did not universally recognize the concept of "germs" at the time. In Semmelweis's day, doctors speculated that illness was a result of "bad air" of some sort, caused by rotting flesh or other organic material.[24] Their thinking was that if you did not have direct contact with foul food or water, you couldn't get sick. Because of this, doctors had no reason to wash their hands in between patients. The idea that material from a dead body could remain on their hands and be passed to the next patient sounded ludicrous.

Semmelweis hadn't discovered germs, but he theorized that "cadaverous material" caused the infections. He demanded that doctors use chlorinated lime — now used in home cleaning solutions — to wash their hands and instruments between patients. His new protocol solved the problem! Deaths in the clinic fell by 90%. At one point in 1847, two months went by without a single patient death.

You would think that Semmelweis's

colleagues would herald him as a hero for his lifesaving discovery. But his theory flew in the face of entrenched medical beliefs at the time. The gentlemanly doctors were insulted by Semmelweis's claim that they had dirty hands or could cause a woman's death.[25]

Dr. Semmelweis later implemented his hand-washing protocol when he became the head physician at an obstetric ward in his hometown of Budapest. Like his clinic in Vienna, the facility was overrun with deadly infections. Due to his strict hand-washing policies, fewer than 1% of patients died from childbed fever over the five years he was in charge.[26] That's amazing. He ushered in the new era of safe maternity care.

Yet Semmelweis still wasn't accepted by his peers. In 1861, he published his greatest work, *The Etiology, Concept and Prophylaxis of Childbed Fever,* which highlighted the backlash. "Most medical lecture halls continue to resound with lectures on epidemic childbed fever and with discourses against my theories," he wrote. "In published medical works, my teachings are either ignored or attacked."

Later, Semmelweis suffered from severe depression and cognitive decline. He became obsessed with childbed fever, unable to talk about anything else. In 1865, he was admitted to a mental institution, where he died. It is speculated that he was beaten by a guard at the facility, causing a wound on his hand which, in a cruel twist of irony, became infected and resulted in his death.

Admitted to a mental asylum and then beaten by a guard? Now I don't feel so bad when trolls online call me names in the comment box that appears below my articles.

Penn Fired Her, the Nobel Committee Gave Her a Prize: Dr. Katalin Karikó

When the Covid pandemic hit, researchers used mRNA technology to rapidly develop a vaccine, and now it's being tested to fight other diseases. But few people know that the technology was developed several years before the pandemic by Dr. Katalin Karikó at the University of Pennsylvania. Using her discovery, the genetic code for making a Covid spike protein was built into the mRNA, just as any code could be set to make any desired protein in the body.

But Dr. Karikó was initially disparaged for the work. In fact, she faced so much opposition that mRNA almost didn't happen.

The University of Pennsylvania moved her office to the outskirts of the campus and cut her pay, and many faculty disdained her, reported the *Wall Street Journal*.[27] She later said doing the work had cost her professionally. "I was demoted four times," she told CNBC.[28]

But Dr. Karikó insisted on continuing.

In her 2023 memoir, she calls the highly acclaimed director of the Gene Therapy Program at Penn one of her early detractors. She said that he demanded she stop speaking Hungarian with her colleagues and refused to use grant money to fund her mRNA projects. She was described as a "difficult" employee by a supervisor for insisting on researching mRNA vaccines.[29] Dr. Karikó said that she was denied basic lab supplies to conduct her experiments, got passed up for a promotion, and was in a dire situation.

Dr. Karikó had difficulty publishing her research in medical journals and getting grants. The idea was too radical for her peers nationally and she didn't have a big title at Penn.[30] She described it as "no grants, no funding, no respect from anyone with any formal power."

However, Dr. David Langer, the chair of neurosurgery at Lenox Hill Hospital in New York City, believed in her. He encouraged the head of neurosurgery at Penn to give her the resources she needed to advance the mRNA vaccine concept. She also had a great collaborator in Dr. Drew Weissman, who helped with her funding. Some believe this was the move that led to the eventual creation of the Covid vaccine. Dr. Weissman also continued the work after the institution had pushed her out.

"Michael Jordan was overlooked by two teams and is the greatest basketball player of all time, [and] Tom Brady was drafted 199th," said Dr. Langer.[31] "The value and the ultimate success of somebody is not always readily apparent, even when it's right in front of your eyes."

It was only *after* the 2023 Nobel Prize was awarded to Dr. Karikó and Dr. Weissman that Penn — which has made a fortune from a patent on Dr. Karikó's work — celebrated the announcement and took credit. All of a sudden, they were proud of Dr. Karikó. The president of Penn called her a "brilliant researcher" who epitomized "scientific inspiration and determination."[32]

Never mind that the institution marginalized her every step of the way. An apology would have been more appropriate. It would have also displayed humility — something that is desperately needed today to help rebuild public trust in institutions.

Every scientist should remember the tumultuous journeys of these innovators. They are an inspiration, ending epidemics and advancing medical care. But the establishment is often resistant to new ideas, marginalizing new ideas with an old fashioned trick — referring to the people who believe in them as "controversial" when they should be called "interesting." (I personally like to refer to people with opposing ideas as "interesting" rather than branding them with a pejorative label.)

Those who hold power are often in their position because they built a career around an idea. They have a vested interest in preserving that idea and reminding people how important it is, even when a better one comes along. Dr. Festinger's principle of cognitive dissonance has been empirically validated by centuries of knowledgeable elites exercising hostility toward new ideas that are not their own. In fact, throughout history and vividly today, new ideas and emerging facts threaten the mental peace of holding on to preexisting beliefs.

Many great scientists came to realize that getting people to believe their ideas would be harder than they had expected. They learned that implementation science (convincing people to adopt new things) is harder than discovery science.

Good leaders are keenly aware that their past achievements will someday be replaced. Rather than fight this inevitable process of progress, they embrace it, even encouraging others to challenge them. Good leadership requires self-awareness and humility, characteristics often in short supply in modern medicine. Leaders who demonstrate these noble character traits encourage others and spur innovation. People also admire leaders who exhibit these qualities. They find them more likable, and are more motivated to work for them. Innovators need to be good leaders to advance their ideas.

The innovators in this chapter were attacked, canceled, demoted, disparaged, defunded, ignored, overlooked, and even burned at the stake! If you're an innovator, don't be surprised if the establishment doesn't welcome your ideas. In fact, it's more likely that they will not.

These great innovators did not give up. They persisted, overcame great barriers, and changed the world. That's inspiring to anyone trying to bring about positive change. We need to keep pushing, stay positive, and support new ideas getting a fair hearing, even if we don't like them.

CHAPTER 11

A Culture of Obedience

The battle for civil discourse

I disapprove of what you say, but I will defend to the death your right to say it.

— Evelyn Beatrice Hall

As I wrote this book, I was asked to give the grand rounds lecture for the Johns Hopkins OB/GYN department. I felt honored. But I noticed a strange question when I filled out the standard paperwork required by the medical school for attendees to claim continuing medical education (CME) credit.

If I am providing recommendations involving clinical medicine, they will be based on evidence that is accepted within the profession of medicine as adequate justification for their indications and contraindications in the care of patients. All scientific research referred to will conform to the generally accepted standard . . .

○ Yes ● No

Of course, I answered "No." After all, my research often challenges assumptions in medicine, using the scientific method: develop a hypothesis, test it, and interpret the findings with an open mind.

Evidently, my "No" answer ruffled some feathers. It generated a lot of confusion and email traffic. Bewildered, the medical education office sent this message off to the event organizer: "Please ask Dr. Makary to explain his answer or was this an error when completing the form?"

Nope, it wasn't an error.

I answered honestly rather than give rote agreement to simply get the bureaucratic form over with. I ended up giving the speech (without any issues), and the head of obstetrics described it as the best speech they've ever had at grand rounds. But the perfunctory form reminded me of just how often we get nudged to go along with the crowd.

Conform or Else

The pressure to conform to conventional thinking has never been stronger. Sometimes it's subtle, and sometimes it's overt. It helps explain why the type of medical misadventures I've been writing about in this book persist.

For example, as scientists, we all need grant funding to do our research. NIH grant applications are reviewed by senior scientists, players in the field who tend to favor proposals that support their older ideas. Some critics argue that's exactly why advancements in cancer, chronic diseases, and biomedicine have been generally stagnant for decades. For example, the return on investment of cancer funding is alarmingly low. The NIH spends approximately $8 billion in taxpayer dollars on cancer research. But the results are rarely impressive. For example, the number one study presented at the big cancer conference showed how an existing chemo drug, given for a type of incurable brain cancer, increased survival by a few months — but cured no one. That's the top breakthrough.

Old scientists entrenched in the field tend to favor legacy ideas when allocating new research dollars. Government research grants are often given for small, incremental research, not big ideas. Some critics of the current system have even suggested that we'd achieve more significant scientific advances if the NIH picked which ideas to fund at random. Or fund some grant applications where only one reviewer scored it highly. Others have suggested that we'd cure more diseases if we took genius researchers and said, here's $10 million, work on whatever you believe is most promising (and it's okay to pivot the research several times along the way — something disallowed under current NIH funding rules).

A similar dynamic whereby the old guard controls academic currency is at play with medical journals and medical societies. In the case of journals, we researchers submit our studies and opinion essays to editors, who are the gatekeepers of what gets read by the broader medical community. They control the airwaves. Editorial boards, which tend to be composed of like-minded friends, hold tremendous power. Many of them never relinquish that power, serving lifetime terms like a European monarch. Because editorial board positions are credentials used in academic promotion, power begets more power. A few editorial boards and medical societies try hard to rotate fresh leadership, but many default to being less inclusive rather than more. It's human nature. Applying Dr. Festinger's theory of cognitive dissonance, those who hold centralized power generally don't like opposing viewpoints.

In 2023, a few of the most powerful medical societies in the U.S. made an unprecedented move to support government actions to silence opposing medical voices. The American Academy of Pediatrics, the American

Medical Association, and other medical societies filed an amicus brief with the U.S. Supreme Court on behalf of the government, supporting government censorship of health information, including opinions expressed by physicians.[1] Their brief argued that the government has "a compelling interest" in combating health misinformation. That could create a dangerous precedent. By this rationale, a doctor who does not recommend a mammogram for a low-risk 40-year-old woman, for example, could possibly be censored at the government's behest.

Many doctors were appalled.

Critics argued that granting the government power to censor speech by doctors — speech that the medical establishment doesn't like — violates not only the letter of the U.S. Constitution's first amendment, but the medical profession's historic liberty to say whatever we believe to be in the best interest of our patients. We have been — and should always be — different from political party patrons who uniformly stick to the same talking points for the purpose of solidarity. For centuries, Harvard's seal and main gate on campus have bannered the institution's motto, "Veritas," which means truth. It does not read "Cancellus."

The battle for freedom of speech among

doctors is also playing out at the state government level. In 2022, California passed a law making a doctor's disagreement with the California Medical Board on certain health recommendations grounds for that doctor to lose their medical license. The law was repealed following outrage by scientists from the University of California San Francisco, Stanford, and other institutions who filed a lawsuit.[2]

What's going on here?

Not allowing doctors to disagree with a state's department of health? Or the recommendations of the American Academy of Pediatrics?

What if the recommendation was based on a study from Harvard's Dana Farber Cancer Institute? In early 2024, the institution along with Brigham and Women's Hospital were forced to retract 6 articles and correct 31 more due to inconsistent or fraudulent data.[3] Under the now repealed 2022 California law, if a California doctor did not believe a recommendation based on one of those fraudulent studies, he or she could lose their medical license.

Doctors need to be able to freely voice their opinions without retribution because some research is flawed.

At Dana-Farber, a total of 29 researchers

were involved, including the institution's CEO. A few of the scientists involved didn't show a lot of humility either. In the investigation, one researcher "expressed regret that he didn't have access to a better version of Photoshop to more convincingly manipulate his images."[4]

Also in early 2024, a researcher at Brigham and Women's was found to have falsified data and plagiarized images in 21 articles. And this was not just some random low-level researcher, it was the vice chair of research of the Brigham and Women's Hospital neurosurgery department.[5] Seven years prior, the hospital had been ordered to pay $10 million after the Department of Justice found it had used "manipulated and falsified information" to obtain NIH funding.[6]

It's not just a bad batch of research studies coming out of Harvard. Over 10,000 medical journal articles were retracted in 2023, setting a new record.[7] Also that year, Stanford University's president resigned following allegations of data manipulation, and the dean of Weill Cornell medical school left his post after similar allegations involving three of his research studies.[8] One was a joint study with Weill Cornell and the Brigham and Women's Hospital that had been cited 178 times.

If all these retractions were found in published articles in the public domain, consider how many more mistakes and fudging errors occur behind the scenes, when researchers collect and tabulate the data. That's one of the big takeaways of Sholto David, a 32-year-old molecular biologist and science journalist who exposed some of the Dana-Farber studies. "Imagine what mistakes might be found in the raw data if anyone was allowed to look!" he wrote.[9]

Well, some are looking. Recently, Dr. John Carlisle, an editor of the medical journal *Anaesthesia,* examined 500 clinical trials and found that a whopping 44% of them contained false data.[10]

Yikes.

Dr. Carlisle conducted his analysis in a smart way. He required researchers submitting their studies to also submit the underlying patient data. He compared the patient data to the data in the article to look for irregularities. His findings were incredible. I had heard of many researchers fudging their data (usually by demanding a low-level person manipulate the numbers to give them certain results), but his study was a reminder that a single study can be wrong. It can also take the medical community down a rabbit hole.

It wasn't just me. Dr. Carlisle's study rattled many people and the blind faith they put in the integrity of what's being published in medical journals.[11] Silencing doctors who disagree removes an important check on the scientific community. We need more debate not more dismissals.

When We Look Under the Hood

Governments have spent billions of dollars since 2002 stockpiling Tamiflu, under the promise that the drug would reduce complications and hospital admissions due to influenza.[12] Dr. Tom Jefferson, an Oxford scientist, not the wealthy U.S. ambassador to France who became the third U.S. president, made a surprising discovery. He reviewed the evidence for Tamiflu for the Cochrane Collaboration organization, a highly respected group of experts who conduct extensive scientific reviews.[13] He went through the clinical notes kept on patients participating in the original Tamiflu trial. Patient-level reports reveal first-hand what happened to each study participant on the drug, but they are typically never made public when a clinical trial is published. In this case, however, the manufacturer, Roche, came under intense public pressure to release the information. Dr. Jefferson's findings rocked the world. He found that Tamiflu wasn't highly effective against the flu — the basis by which governments had stockpiled the drug. In fact, it barely worked.

It turns out that not even the coauthors of the original study on Tamiflu had seen the patient-level reports. So the one time that the world medical community got a peek into what patient-level reports actually found, it changed the conclusions of the trial. I was amazed to learn that it's typical for patient-level data in clinical trials to be kept private. Imagine what they might tell us if patient-level reports were routinely made public.[14] Imagine how many other trials would have different results.

Dr. Elisabeth Bik, a microbiologist and microbiome expert, conducted a similar investigation. She began noticing fraudulent pictures in journal articles, specifically photos of genetic tests that looked doctored. She screened scientific articles to see if they had numerical inconsistencies, manipulated images, or implausible results. In an analysis of 20,000 research articles, she found manipulated photographs in 1 in every 25 of the studies.[15] Some of these studies were used by researchers to obtain taxpayer dollars via large NIH grants.

If we're seeing this much bad data just in

published studies, imagine how many other ways research can be fudged. Dr. Bik is now using AI software to identify additional doctored images. But the solution is not just using AI to police publishing errors; we need a system that funds repeating research studies to confirm the results.

The revelations of manipulated data should make us all see the shortcomings of the peer review process. It's an added layer of review, but not an end-all seal of approval that a study is trustworthy.

"Peer review has never been the gold standard or *Good Housekeeping* Seal of Approval . . . that journals and scientists and universities and federal agencies want us to think it is," said Dr. Ivan Oransky, co-founder of the watchdog blog *Retraction Watch*.[16]

He's right. Sometimes a peer review is detailed and represents a truly independent assessment, but most of the time it's the same as a comment box below an online news article. In fact, comment boxes may be better because the author is rarely anonymous. Most peer reviewers are anonymous. Medical journals have an odd tradition of keeping the names of reviewers secret from the authors of a study. If they were truly dedicated to addressing cronyism, they would flip it. Reviewers should review studies while blinded to who authored them. That would help ensure an objective, nonpolitical assessment of the merits of any study. A few medical journals have recently started doing this.

I have also noted that many times what gets published depends on who you know. I've had several editors or leaders in specialty groups ask me to submit an article to their journal or medical conference, saying they'll see to it that it gets accepted. That's not a good way to advance research. These behind-the-scenes practices crowd out new ideas and sometimes explains why research seems stagnant, despite the massive societal investment.

The primary role of medical journals is to filter what research doctors read. You can imagine how powerful that gatekeeper role is, and how it could be weaponized if journals lose their objectivity. Personally, I've always found it strange that newspapers, like the *Washington Post,* would "endorse" a political candidate. That's why it's even more disturbing for a medical journal to do so. Throughout its 208-year history, the *New England Journal* remained staunchly nonpartisan.[17] But four weeks before the 2020 presidential election, that suddenly changed. The medical journal essentially endorsed a candidate.[18] The sharply worded article was signed by its 34 editors. The science journal *Nature* did the same thing.[19] The problem here is not with who they chose, it's the issue of getting into politics. It's a new precedent that has many doctors concerned about who's controlling the biggest spigot of health information.

Medical journals should return to their centuries-old tradition of not giving out political endorsements.

The Silencing

In 2022, my friend and former Baltimore health commissioner Dr. Leana Wen was invited to speak on a panel on bullying and harassment at the American Public Health Association's annual conference. Even though she was a card-carrying supporter of Covid mandates, some of her views had somewhat changed by 2022. She suggested lifting some Covid restrictions and spoke about individual responsibility. "This is our new normal — one that's based on individuals being thoughtful about their own risks and the risks they pose to others," she wrote.

But the public health ruling class does not tolerate dissenting opinions on sacred cow topics. More than 600 public health academics and national leaders signed a letter demanding that she be removed from the meeting and not allowed to speak. Although she did not manipulate data in a clinical trial or Photoshop images in a Harvard publication, in the eyes of the public health academic community, she had done something far worse: She had expressed an opinion different from theirs. She had committed a thought crime.

The intense national pressure to excommunicate Dr. Wen worked. She did not speak at the conference panel on bullying. Instead, she was bullied out of the conference by the experts in the field. The news was deeply disappointing to me. I always enjoyed my conversations with Dr. Wen. Even though we had different views on public health topics facing this country, she was reliably polite and friendly, offering the kind of civility this country desperately needs to debate difficult issues. She and I guest-lectured in a class together where we presented different viewpoints. She was a class act.

Bothered by the hostility of the public health establishment toward Dr. Wen, I spoke with the executive director of the American Public Health Association and asked him why he didn't allow different points of view at his conference. He simply invited me to attend the conference.

I looked into attending but soon discovered that it would not be possible. The large academic conference only allowed researchers to attend if they had received three or more Covid vaccine shots. After being elected to the National Academy of Medicine, I got barred from attending their national conference for the same reason: I had only received two Covid shots — an insufficient number to attend for the conference. This, despite having natural immunity from a previous Covid infection months before, something I described in a study my team conducted.[20] Our study, which demonstrated high antibody levels from people who recovered from Covid, was censored from social media platforms. However, the study was well received by doctors. Doctors used it to tailor their Covid booster recommendations in low-risk individuals. A year later, *JAMA* listed the study on its website as the third most discussed article they had published in 2022.[21]

Freedom of speech is not designed for easy speech — speech that is welcomed by the majority because it affirms their beliefs. It's designed to protect speech that is uncomfortable — speech that challenges groupthink. Today, more than ever, organized medicine is finding ways to limit and stifle scientific debate. Some of these ways are subtle, such as inviting like-minded people to editorial boards, committees, and conferences. Other methods of suppression are overt, such as hospital communications departments telling doctors that they can't talk to the media without going through them — a policy that American doctors share with doctors in North Korea. Dozens of leading medical experts have privately told me that someone from their hospital's communications department staff has called them to give them a hard time, or even bully them, after they say something in a media interview that the hospital didn't like. Americans don't want to hear from medical propogandists, they want to hear from doctors speaking freely.

Time and time again, institutions and organized medicine have kept the dissenting opinions of highly credentialed doctors hush-hush, creating an illusion of consensus. But the track record of organizations that do this is not very good. Just look at how the medical establishment performed on the giant health recommendations detailed in this book. Now more than ever, we need doctors and scientists to speak honestly on the biggest health issues of our day. We need civil discourse.

The cancellation of Dr. Wen did not fall along partisan lines. While nearly every academic public health leader considers themself to be politically liberal, Dr. Wen is hardly a conservative. She was a Democratic political appointee and later served as the CEO of Planned Parenthood. She is now a public health researcher at George Washington University and a columnist for the *Washington Post*. It's ironic that universities claim to believe in inclusion and racial, ethnic, and age diversity but, oddly, ideological diversity is excluded.

The *Wall Street Journal* editorial board weighed in on the American Public Health Association conference incident. "Apparently public-health experts also can't be allowed to make their own decisions about whether to listen to Dr. Wen," the board wrote.[22]

It's not just the American Public Health Association. Many national societies tend to become fiefdoms. I remember attending the annual American College of Surgeons conference as a surgical resident. I attended a panel discussion on pancreas surgery, composed of a few big names in the field. I was blown away by the opportunity to hear them and meet them. After all, I had read their writings for years. But then I went back the following year. It was the same people on the panel, making similar remarks. Over the next ten years, there were a few other experts that rotated through the panel, but essentially it always featured the same legacy experts. It's no wonder this group downplayed the innovation of minimally invasive pancreas surgery that reduced postoperative pain and infection rates. They personally didn't know how to perform these operations.

I know many doctors who have given up submitting research to medical conferences or journals because they are so highly curated by a small group of people, and they aren't interested in playing the political game needed to get their work published. We are scientists, not socialites. Dr. Ahmet Baschat, a senior Johns Hopkins colleague who is boarded in three medical specialties and a highly accomplished researcher, is one of the critics. "There's a lot of publication politics," Dr. Baschat told me. "I don't like going to conferences anymore because it's a sales show by a small group of people."

Today, the control of the medical ruling class to limit debate has never been tighter. People are labeled quickly for holding certain views or presenting new ones. Last year, the National Academy of Medicine had on the top of the first page of its application for membership a box to check if the candidate for consideration has an interest in climate change. I'm a believer in climate change, but is that how we want to screen medical doctors for membership? In 2023, the president of a leading surgical society dared to express his personal views *questioning* affirmative action in surgery. Rather than disagree with his viewpoint, the society's leadership excoriated him, a shot across the bow to anyone who dares question conventional wisdom supporting affirmative action hiring in surgery.[23] A University of Pittsburgh cardiologist was similarly removed from leadership for questioning affirmative action. What ever happened to simply disagreeing and presenting counterpoints? The environment around certain issues in medicine has become toxic.

The Principal Has a Paddle

Earlier this year, Dr. Richard Baron, the CEO of the powerful American Board of Internal Medicine (ABIM), a privately-owned monopoly, came to give a speech at Johns Hopkins. He did not talk about the latest cures for cancer or heart disease. His talk was entitled "Protecting the Legitimacy of Medical Expertise: Combating Misinformation in Medicine," a speech in which he argued for a small priesthood of physicians to delineate which medical opinions doctors should be allowed to express in public. He highlighted the association's new decertify program, aimed at removing the board certification of any doctor that does not agree with ABIM leadership positions on certain medical controversies. (For context, this board will also revoke certification if a doctor does not pay them $220 each year. Imagine if the college you graduated from told you to pay them each year and take a quiz to keep your college degree. That's what the American Board of Medical Specialties is doing to nearly all board-certified physicians.) The ABIM and several other medical boards issued a statement in 2021 that doctors have an ethical duty "to share information" that is "consensus-driven" and if they disagree, the board will put their board certification at risk.[24] His talk did *not* mention one of the greatest needs in medicine today: civil discourse. Following the Covid pandemic, I know of doctors at the hospital who are not speaking to each other over differences in their medical opinions. We should rise above the noise and engage in the hard work of ensuring civility rather than a police state to crack down on scientific thought crimes.

It's not just in medicine. In 2024, Harvard economics professor Dr. Roland Fryer was told not to publish his 2017 study that showed that while police were more likely to show excessive force against racial minorities, they were less likely *to shoot them* compared to white suspects.[25] Colleagues told him he should publish the first part, which they liked — but not the second part. But he decided to publish all the results. In an interview with journalist Bari Weiss of the *Free Press,* he explained how after that, his life became "hell." He immediately became the subject of an internal investigation at Harvard and was suspended for two years without pay. He was not fired, because he was tenured — the youngest Black tenured professor at Harvard. "People lose their minds when they don't like the result," he told Weiss. (Dr. Fryer's boss who suspended him, Dr. Claudine Gay, would later be named president of Harvard, and then be forced to resign due to plagiarism.)[26]

Societies are defined by what speech they do not permit.

If we expel doctors who disagree with establishment organizations like the American Academy of Pediatrics, then doctors who challenged their peanut abstinence recommendation could have been excommunicated. If the California law had been in place 10 to 20 years ago, Dr. Gideon Lack, whose research led to overturning the peanut abstinence recommendation, would have been regarded not as an innovator, but as a fugitive.

Shutting Down Debate

Universities are supposed to be the last bastion of free speech. In fact, many pride themselves in this mission. But ironically, America's elite universities have shut down all debate around some of the biggest issues of our day. During the Covid pandemic, Harvard, Stanford, Penn, University of California San Francisco (UCSF), Brown, and Johns Hopkins had zero debates on Covid policy. I mention those particular institutions because that's where I have friends in leadership who confirmed that to be true.

The first debate at the Massachusetts Institute of Technology (MIT) took place after the pandemic, on February 27, 2024, on the topic of the school's Covid vaccine booster mandate. Many doctors believe that a young healthy male student who recently had Covid does not need a booster, and getting one would add the risk of myocarditis, which occurs in approximately 1 in 2,000 young men. One of these doctors is UCSF's Dr. Vinay Prasad, who has written more than 20 peer-reviewed scientific studies on Covid. He presented this view on

MIT's debate stage. He described the many students who attended the debate as highly engaged and open-minded! Many thanked him for his perspective.

People are hungry for civil discourse.

A smaller debate was held at UCSF after the pandemic, but during the pandemic, the hot issues of prolonged school closures, yearslong hospital visitation bans, and cloth mask mandates for toddlers (except when they were eating or napping at day care) had zero debate at America's elite universities. Evidently, allowing students and faculty to hear expert opinions that deviated from the administration's would have been too much for them to handle. But as we saw in chapter 6, "Bad Blood," when health officials dismiss good questions simply to protect the faith in health institutions, it can result in disaster. In the case of sidelining people who questioned the risk of HIV in the blood supply, protecting the Red Cross brand at any expense resulted in the death of most Americans with severe hemophilia.

It's okay to be wrong. In science, when people get things wrong when little information is available, they are being human. But when they make absolutist claims for years that go against overwhelming medical evidence simply to protect an institution's or political party's brand, they are propogandists.

A Bright Spot

The Royal Society in London is perhaps the most prestigious scientific association in the world. Its rich history of promoting an open forum of ideas began with Sir Isaac Newton, who served as its first president. The Royal Society boasts that its members are elected based purely on scientific merit, not academic titles or who they know. The Royal Society ushered in scientists like Albert Einstein and Steven Hawking, who challenged conventional thinking. As a testament to its mission to do just that, the Royal Society has published articles that many people did not like, such as Benjamin Franklin's kite experiment. To this day, the Royal Society has continued to promote groundbreaking work on antibiotic-resistant bacteria and theoretical physics.

At the core of the Royal Society's mission is its motto, *Nullius in verba,* which means "Take nobody's word for it." The words are prominently ingrained at the entrance to its building. Further, the Royal Society states that its motto "is an expression of the determination of Fellows to withstand the domination of authority and to verify all statements by an appeal to facts determined by experiment." Amen.

Wading Against the Current

Throughout my career in medicine, I've focused on studying topics I couldn't stop thinking about — our blind spots as a profession. Blind spots form not because we have diabolical people in health care. On the contrary, we have good people working in a bad system — a system we didn't design. It's a system we inherited. Blind spots exist not because smart people are malicious. They occur when we have an intense focus on our work. In the case of medicine, it's the altruistic focus on taking care of sick people.

My curiosity began as a medical student. Blind spots seemed to be a treasure trove for scientific discovery. I took an interest in the giant issues in medicine that we didn't talk about but should be talking about. Naysayers would often discourage me from pursuing these topics, though many eventually came full circle.

I wanted to work on important issues that were underappreciated and underfunded. My journey challenging medicine's groupthink and it's deeply held assumptions has been an adventure. Allow me to tell you a little bit about it.

I quickly learned that the dangers of tobacco were the number one rallying cry of the medical community. The data were clear. But our strategy seemed focused on demeaning users of tobacco. We shamed them, referring to them not as human beings struggling with tobacco addiction but as "smokers." Every single correspondence between health professionals began with that. "We have a 45-year-old smoker here with an ingrown toenail," we'd say. Or "I'm sending a 52-year-old smoker up to the fourth floor for an X-ray of his knee." It was our attempt to label and brand a class of people, many of whom avoided doctors.

Yet there was an issue no one seemed to be talking about: Hospitals and medical schools were funding the tobacco companies by investing a portion of their large endowments in them. It was a massive blind spot, a moral failure. With the help of my professor Dr. Ichiro Kawachi, I wrote an article in *JAMA* calling on hospitals, medical schools, and health insurance companies to divest their tobacco stocks.[27] One person who ran a university endowment said to me, "You don't understand how it works, it's not that simple." Dr. Kawachi and I were repeatedly told divestment would never happen.

But over the next 20 years, many institutions

in health care did exactly that, including most of the top universities with medical schools in the country. When the string of divestments occurred, I recalled the hospital expert who had told me it would never happen, and the sage advice of one of my mentors who told me, "Ninety percent of success is just figuring out who's full of B.S."

As a resident I was struck by another big issue no one was talking about: the high number of people harmed by preventable medical errors. I had witnessed people dying not from the disease that brought them to care, but from the care itself. I personally made mistakes from being foisted into situations above my level of training, from poor judgment when experiencing sleep deprivation, and from breakdowns in communication. The most dangerous procedure in the emergency department was a patient handoff — when one doctor or nurse hands off a patient to another doctor or nurse, summarizing their medical issues with a quick description. Some of those errors haunted me. At one point, I took on a cold and robotic personality to cope, which also affected my personal relationships outside the hospital. But in talking to my co-residents, I realized nearly everyone was experiencing the same things.

A rare few spoke of the epidemic of medical errors; they included doctors at different institutions such as Drs. David Bates, Lucian Leape, and Don Berwick. I read their articles and met with each of them, affirming my suspicion that there was an alarming epidemic happening right under our noses. They estimated the death toll to be as high as 100,000 deaths per year. These doctors believed that patient safety should be a science and encouraged me to pursue it as my academic focus. My dean told me I was wasting my time. A few mentors were supportive, but the old guard said it was not a real science, pointing out how it was career suicide because I would never get an NIH grant to study how to prevent medical errors. Instead, they insisted that all surgical residents spend a year or two working in a laboratory.

I decided to take a risk and study patient safety.

I did studies on nontechnical skills like teamwork and communication. With a few colleagues, we measured safety culture with validated surveys. Then one day, my mentor Dr. Peter Pronovost encouraged me to come up with a checklist for surgery, based on one he had created for the ICU. I drafted a few questions, modeled after a cockpit checklist pilots use before flying a plane, and began using it before my operations. The first question was: What are the names and roles of each person in the operating room? Then we confirmed the patient's name, the operation we were doing, and the correct side of the operation. We added a few questions to ensure we had the equipment and backup we needed and, voilà, we had a surgery checklist.[28]

"No one is going to use this," one of my surgical colleagues told me. Another colleague who tried it told me, "I feel like this is the Mickey Mouse Club." But then I asked my colleagues to try it for several months so we could study its impact on safety. We found that the use of a surgical checklist improved patient safety culture and improved patient outcomes.[29,30]

After I published articles detailing our experience using a surgery checklist at Johns Hopkins, the WHO invited me to present the checklist to a newly convened committee. The committee, led by Dr. Atul Gawande, loved it and quickly put the WHO seal on it. The checklist I developed became known as the WHO surgery checklist and was soon posted on the wall of every operating room in the world. When I was a resident, no one used a checklist before doing surgery.

Today, it's standard of care. It's been estimated that in the first year the checklist was widely used worldwide, it saved more lives than the incremental benefit of the newest chemotherapy that same year. At no point did the NIH fund this type of work.

I went on to write a book on the topic called *Unaccountable,* calling for hospitals to publicly report their rates of medical errors known as "never events," a list of things that should never happen in a hospital. In the book I called on hospitals to publicly report their infection rates, readmission rates, and other quality measures. Again, I was told it would never happen. Medical elites from health care organizations told me it was a pipe dream. Within a few years of the book becoming a *New York Times* bestseller, Medicare began requiring public reporting of all of the above quality metrics.

Another striking blind spot I noticed in medicine was understanding frailty. Some old people were healthy but frail. Others had comorbidities but were non-frail. I decided to conduct a clinical trial to see what predicted surgical outcome better — the level of frailty, as measured by a five-point index, or more traditional preoperative tests like cardiac testing. Some highly decorated researchers nationally told me this was a soft study. However, the research revealed that frailty was *the* most powerful predictor of surgical outcomes, more predictive than traditional preoperative testing.[31] Today, frailty is recognized as a domain of health that influences surgical decision-making.

Another blind spot my research took on was the carbon footprint of hospitals. Hospitals tend to be the second biggest producers of waste in a community. We published an article in 2011 encouraging hospitals to use more efficient lighting, reduce hazardous waste by educating people about which wastebasket to use for different items, and other green practices.[32] Fast-forward ten years, many hospitals have adopted these practices.

Another blind spot was how certain hospitals that we have come to love were beginning to engage in price gouging and predatory billing. I did a study to document how prevalent this practice was and published a report in *JAMA* showing that one third of hospitals sue patients who can't afford to pay their bill.[33] They sue them to garnish their paychecks, most commonly from their job at Walmart. In one town of about 28,000 people, their beloved community hospital had filed 25,000 lawsuits against residents. In another town, they sued the judge by accident! I wrote about my team's research in my book *The Price We Pay*. You'll never get hospitals to change, I heard again and again. Within three years, many hospitals responded to the media attention brought about by our work and shut down the practice of suing patients. Overall hospital lawsuits against patients dropped by 80%, a finding we documented in a follow-up *JAMA* article.[34]

We are now creating billing quality measures so that hospitals can be rated on a 1- to 5-star scale on their billing quality, allowing consumers to be informed and empowered.[35] The goal is that transparency will enable the market to reward hospitals that are fair, reasonable, and merciful with their billing practices.

When some people had read the thesis of *The Price We Pay,* calling for a requirement for all hospitals to post cash prices for shoppable services, they told me it would never happen. Within two years of the book coming out, many members of Congress and White House officials had read the book and invited me in to discuss details of the proposal. Within a year, a White House executive order was signed, and today hospitals are making their prices public. The idea was so nonpolitical that both Republican and Democrat administrations, as well as the courts, have upheld the new law. It's been bipartisan because transparency is an American value.

For many of these endeavors our research team at Johns Hopkins has taken on, people told us we were wasting our time. I was often excluded from conferences that considered only laboratory research or clinical trials to be real research. Even so, each area of our team's work has had a national or global impact far greater than I could have imagined.

Fortunately, in each case there was a minority of leaders who recognized the problem and helped advance the work. We were successful because of their willingness to consider nonconventional research on topics off the NIH's radar.

One such doctor was Dr. Zubin Damania, perhaps the greatest influencer in medicine today (with over a billion collective views on his various media platforms). A Stanford-trained physician, Dr. Damania has used his unique megaphone to interview experts and discuss important blind spots that the medical establishment doesn't discuss.[36]

In addition, a group of us started the medical news website Sensible Medicine, led today by Drs. Vinay Prasad, Adam Cifu, and John Mandrola — three leading doctors with impeccable credentials. The articles challenge modern medical dogma that pops up daily in medical journals and current events. The pieces challenge medical societies, conference announcements, Big Pharma, and decisions at the FDA, NIH, and CDC in real time. We were told it would be impossible to standup such an independent medical news analysis service without taking advertising revenue, but, I'm happy to report once again that the naysayers were wrong. The website now has over 80,000 readers and growing. Many readers are physicians. Sensible Medicine has never accepted a dollar from a Pharma company or institution. The site has created accountability for the medical establishment, including medical societies and journals. Some articles have been read by half a million people. What we were told was impossible is now changing medicine.

At the opening of this chapter, I showed you the standard form on which I was asked to confirm that my work was "accepted within the profession." In nearly every research endeavor of my career, the idea we studied was *not* initially accepted within the profession.

But then, eventually, it became accepted. Today, when I meet with students and doctors who are passionate about addressing blind spots in medicine but are discouraged from doing so by the establishment, I share my journey with them. I also remind them that the medical field needs fresh new approaches. It needs renaissance thinkers, not workers who just obediently recite catechisms without questioning them. The key is to have the humility to evolve your thinking as you learn along the way.

We Need Ben Franklins

Modern medicine needs people who think big. Renaissance thinkers, like Ben Franklin. Franklin made dozens of scientific contributions, including inventions ranging from the lightning rod and the Pennsylvania stove to a flexible bladder catheter and bifocal glasses. He designed city sanitation projects and proposed ways infections could spread indoors, defying conventional thinking. He was not just a brilliant mind, he was a doer. A fierce critic of slavery, he was a champion of democracy, and a bestselling author. He co-founded America's first hospital, Pennsylvania Hospital. But today's medical culture crushes the creativity of Ben Franklin thinkers. In fact, if a doctor has broad interests, the system insists that they surrender them to focus on one. Doctors cannot get

NIH funding, and hence build an academic career, unless they obediently stay on a narrow research path, proposing incremental steps instead of bold ideas. And if a doctor's ideas cross disciplinary lines, the NIH says we can't support you. Ben Franklin would likely be stifled in academics today.

But medicine today needs more Ben Franklin thinkers.

A New Generation

I'm encouraged by a new generation of health professionals who are willing to get off the hamster wheel of medicine. They aspire to be renaissance thinkers, not cogs on a corporate wheel. They have no allegiance to tradition when it conflicts with an opportunity to make a difference. Social justice is a generational value, and to do something bigger they are willing to explore hybrid medical careers.

Many are starting companies or joining start-ups that are disrupting the way medicine is delivered. Together, we're asking new questions. For example:

- Can diabetes be more effectively treated with a cooking class than by prescribing insulin?
- Can we lower high blood pressure by

improving sleep quality and reducing stress instead of throwing antihypertensive medications at people?

- Can we discuss school lunch programs, not just bariatric surgery and Ozempic?
- Can we treat the epidemic of loneliness by fostering communities instead of simply prescribing antidepressants?
- Can we study the impact of body inflammation on health?
- Can we study environmental exposures that cause cancer, not just the chemotherapy to treat it?

They are even willing to ask the deep and uncomfortable question we often need to ask: Is something we assume to help actually doing more harm than good? *Are we burning the village to save it?*

A new generation of health professionals are nonconformists. They are refusing to kiss the ring of medical oligarchs, and instead are teaming up with creative people to redesign medical care. They are starting new businesses, exploring new areas like the microbiome and food-as-medicine. They are laser-focused on fixing our broken system.

Chronic diseases are the leading cause of death in the U.S. and consume a majority of the $4.5 trillion we spend on health care.

The current reactionary, siloed, Whac-A-Mole health care system isn't working. Most American adults take four or more prescription medications regularly, making the U.S. the most medicated population in the world. We need to try new approaches to health. We need fresh ideas.

The Future

Modern medicine, and society in general, are now fighting an intellectual civil war about whether the scientific method or consensus opinion should regulate inquiry. The powerful nudges that I describe in the opening of this chapter are a small sample of how the battle continues to be played out every day.

It's hardly a new struggle. Throughout history, civilizations have swung from open-mindedness to cancel culture. In the United States, we must now ask if scientific inquiry is exempt from our democratic values, or if civility in open discourse is a value we truly espouse.

Today's great thinkers, writers, and journalists, from both sides of the political aisle, are pointing out how we need to be aware how power begets more power and groupthink can smother good ideas. As Noam Chomsky described it, "If you don't believe in freedom of speech for people you disagree with, you don't believe in freedom of speech at all."

Open debate and a discussion of the merits of data over dogma make for a stronger society, more civility, and a faster rate of medical discovery.

CHAPTER 12

IMAGINE

What else are we getting wrong?

There are in fact two things, science and opinion; the former begets knowledge, the latter ignorance.

— Hippocrates

If the modern medical establishment got so many major health recommendations wrong over the last few decades, it raises an unsettling question: What are we getting wrong today?

Unfortunately, medical dogma may be more prevalent today than in the past because intolerance for different opinions is on the rise, and medical authority is more centralized.

Many of today's medical practices are not supported by good studies. A study by Drs. Vinay Prasad, Adam Cifu, and colleagues found that 40% of accepted practices did not hold up when rigorously tested.[1]

When Bob Marley noted a discoloration

on his foot, his doctors told him it was likely a sports injury. Conventional thinking was that black people don't get melanoma. We now recognize that teaching for what it really was — medical dogma. The singer went on to die of melanoma at age 36.

It's okay to use clinical wisdom to fill the gaps where research has yet to be done. But recommendations lacking proper scientific support should be recognized as opinion, not scientific evidence. A former editor of *JAMA* once told me that 60% of what we as physicians do in medicine is discretionary. In other words, a lot of what we do is not supported by good scientific evidence.

The medical profession should be funding studies to address these gaps, but it's doing the opposite. Most research today is concentrated in the pharmaceutical space because that's where funding is abundant. Studies that lead to a drug's approval are rarely repeated — for fear they might not yield the same favorable results. And studies on food and lifestyle changes are rarely supported by industry or government agencies. As a result, we spend billions on new drugs and blood tests, but very little to study how food affects body inflammation, nutrition, and the microbiome.

My research team at Johns Hopkins and I actively watch new ideas being introduced in medical journals, at conferences, and in the media. We see one of two reactions. Some receive innovative ideas with curiosity and objectivity while others become territorial and tribal.

In this chapter, we'll explore ten current medical practices that are based on assumptions that have not yet been fully or properly studied. You probably have preconceived ideas about what a future study might reveal about each of them, but let's agree that in the absence of good evidence, current viewpoints are opinions.

Let's agree to be open-minded. If someone calls their view on one of these examples "evidence-based" when there is no good evidence, they are either ignorant or purposefully deceptive. If Dr. Festinger were alive, he'd likely explain that misrepresenting one's opinion as evidence-based is simply a coping mechanism to satisfy one's cognitive dissonance.

Given the number of major health recommendations that have been reversed once properly studied, imagine how many more things we recommend today might be reserved if they were properly studied. *Imagine.*

1. Fluoride in Drinking Water

Fluoride kills bacteria in the mouth that causes cavities, which is why it was added to the water supply. But fluoride may also be killing bacteria in the microbiome.

And altering the microbiome isn't the only potential problem with putting fluoride in drinking water. It may be affecting our intelligence. A 2019 study in *JAMA Pediatrics* reported "maternal exposure to higher levels of fluoride during pregnancy was associated with lower IQ scores" in young children. Fluoride gets transferred through a mother's blood to her baby. It accumulates in brain regions involved in learning and memory, and it alters proteins and neurotransmitters in the central nervous system.

In the past, dentists saw research suggesting that fluoridation of water reduces cavities. As a result, they made it a public health cause. It seemed simple. They were also using the one hammer they had to address the problem they see the most. They pushed for it everywhere, in the U.S. and in poor countries around the world. Today, fluoride is added to the drinking water of about 66% of U.S. residents. It's added to the water of 38% of Canadian residents and 3% of European residents.

Experts in the areas of microbiome and pediatric neurodevelopment tend to have a more nuanced view. And as an aside, it says something to me that the two dentists I trust the most both use toothpaste without fluoride and have expensive systems in their homes to defluoridate their water.

When I took a hard look at the studies, the data to support fluoride in drinking water to prevent cavities is flimsier than people realize. A Cochrane Collaboration review found that there's "very little contemporary evidence" evaluating the effectiveness of water fluoridation to prevent cavities. Most studies were done before 1975 and had study-design issues. In addition, the studies did not consider the increasingly common use of fluoride toothpaste and other measures that may reduce cavities. In addition, many countries that have not added fluoride in their drinking water have also seen reduced cavity rates.[2]

Another argument that has been used to add fluoride to the water supply is that it can kill bacteria in water treatment plants, like chlorine does. The city of Washington, D.C., does this, even as they also pour raw sewage from the city into the local river. Here's a radical idea to make our drinking water safer and cleaner: Stop pouring raw sewage into the local river that provides our city's water.

Is fluoridation of water a great public health achievement, or is it possibly harmful? All I know for certain is that if someone tells you that fluoridation of the water supply is entirely safe and essential for public health, that is an opinion, not a fact.

The non-dental effects of fluoride deserve more rigorous study. If the data go against decades-long dogma supporting fluoridated water, fluoride may be doing more harm than good. Even as the CDC calls the fluoridation of drinking water to prevent cavities "one of ten great public health achievements of the twentieth century,"[3] we should be open to reversing this practice.

2. "Marijuana is harmless"

The belief that marijuana is safe and definitely not a gateway drug looms large in society today, even among some doctors. Two dozen states have legalized recreational use of marijuana, as of 2023,[4] and its use has become mainstream. But could it be that we are convincing ourselves what we want to be true?

The marijuana of today is not the marijuana of hippies from decades ago. In the last several years, manufacturers got smart and now, compared to the 1970s, it includes ten times as much *tetrahydrocannabinol,* the psychoactive component better known as THC.[5] It also may be more harmful to adolescents than to adults,[6] which is why an adult's anecdotal experience should not become the basis of a firm scientific position on the issue in children. The developing adolescent brain may be more susceptible to long-term damage.

A study by Swedish researchers found that young people who used marijuana had up to a sixfold increased risk of developing schizophrenia compared to those who did not. Other studies have found that as many as 1 in 10 young people who use marijuana will develop psychotic symptoms later in life. In a review by Ann Abouseif at Harvard University, she found "an apparent correlation between early cannabis use and several neurological and psychological adverse consequences in adolescence and continuing into adulthood."[7]

Marijuana also seems to be worsening our teenagers' mental health crisis. A McGill–Oxford meta-analysis found a 37% increased risk of depression and more than a 300% increase risk in suicidal ideation among adolescents who used cannabis.[8]

Marijuana may also affect intelligence.

One study suggested that an earlier onset and frequent use during adolescence was directly associated with declines in verbal IQ and executive function tasks, such as trial and error learning and conditional association learning.[9]

Finally, it's well known in the field of cardiology that marijuana use increases the risk of heart attack and strokes — a 25% and 42% increase respectively, according to a 2024 study published in *JAMA*.[10]

Between the risk of psychosis, increased rates of anxiety and depression, and cardiovascular disease, "harmless" is not the word I would use to describe the drug. Sure, it may be less lethal than cocaine, but it's not exactly an organic kale salad.

People should be aware of these risks. Afterall, marijuana is the most common drug used by adolescents.[11]

I'll acknowledge that there are *underappreciated* health benefits to THC, the active ingredient in marijuana. I've seen patients with Crohn's disease and terminal cancer benefit from "medical marijuana." But that doesn't mean it's safe for young developing minds.

Another big question is: Is marijuana a gateway drug? What blows me away is how many people have strong opinions that it's not, without any robust data to support their position. An Australian study that followed nearly 2,000 students who used marijuana for a decade concluded that "Occasional adolescent cannabis use predicts later drug use and later education problems."[12] Another study that followed young people even longer found similar results.[13]

Drug abuse and addiction is a major root problem in society (incidentally, the drug with the highest abuse rate and death toll in America — alcohol — receives little attention). It drives crime, ruins familes, and kills more than 100,000 Americans each year. You would think that people would be open to solutions rather than insisting passionately that marijuana is not a gateway drug.

There is also an economic argument that legalizing marijuana kneecaps the cartels. While that debate is outside the scope of this book, consider this reality: An estimated 80% of marijuana sold in the U.S. is grown illegally[14] by cartels and Chinese organized crime groups operating large farms in places like California, Oklahoma, and Kentucky.[15,16] Some traffic in their own workers — a modern form of slavery on U.S. soil today. In fact, Humboldt County, California, a mecca of illegal marijuana farms, has one of the highest rates of murder and missing persons in the state. One rural California sheriff told the *Louisville Courier Journal,* "I'm fighting a dragon with a needle."

The prevailing (popular) view on how to tackle America's drug crisis is to increase law enforcement and/or legalize drugs. Another approach, that does not exclude other tactics, is to lower demand.

If we are going to be objective, we need to stop saying that marijuana is harmless and not a gateway drug. The truth is that the available evidence does not support those opinions.

3. Tylenol for Fevers

As a resident sleeping in the call room, I got woken up many times for calls that went something like this: "Your patient has a fever of [temperature]. I gave Tylenol, is there anything else you'd like to do?"

It was a given. It seemed like every single hospitalized patient with a fever got dosed with Tylenol.

For decades, modern medicine regarded a fever as a complication that must be universally treated with medication. But that was and continues to be medical dogma. Several studies have suggested that treating fevers may prolong illness. That's because fevers are the body's way of naturally fighting an infection. A Johns Hopkins study of children with chickenpox infection found that those who had their fever medicated had a longer duration of illness compared to those whose fever was not medicated.[17] Other studies have similarly shown that infections last longer when a fever is lowered with medications like Tylenol.[18]

What's going on here? An elevated body temperature may help fight off some bacteria and viruses or bolster the immune system; both mechanisms are suggested in the medical literature.[19,20] Many pediatricians I respect told me how treating fevers with medication should be reserved only for occasions when the condition causes discomfort or pain. There are no hard and fast rules based on the exact temperature number. Some children can run around and be unbothered by a high temperature while others are miserable from even a low-grade temperature. It's not wrong to treat a fever, but the decision should be individualized rather than universal. If a child is uncomfortable, treating the fever may be the humane thing to do.

Ironically, before the era of antibiotics, doctors induced fevers in people in an attempt to fight off infections. Now we've come full circle. Yet the dogma to treat all fevers with Tylenol looms large. Some still try to bat down every temperature elevation like a game of Whac-A-Mole. A 2021 study estimated that 90% of children and half of pregnant mothers[21] take Tylenol or similar fever-lowering medications. Some doctors have expressed concerns about the high utilization of these medications. In 2021, Duke researchers published a warning in a study titled "Paracetamol (Acetaminophen) Use in Infants and Children Was Never Shown to Be Safe for Neurodevelopment."[22] In other words, these drugs may have affects we have not fully appreciated.

In pediatrics the dogma was fueled by fear that a fever could cause a seizure. But in the rare cases when it does, it's the *rate of increase* of the fever, not its peak temperature number, that is implicated in seizures.

Occasionally, a patient will tell me they had a fever but didn't take anything for it because they don't like to take drugs. I smile and tell them it's okay. In fact, it may be wise.

4. The Holy Grail of Early Cancer Detection

One of the big rages in medicine today is a blood test called a liquid biopsy which looks for different types of cancer. The most popular version, the new Multi-Cancer Early Detection Galleri blood test, is made by a company called Grail. Questioning the benefit of this test is hard. After all, who dares to oppose "early cancer detection"? That looks bad. It's like being opposed to food for babies.

The problem is that the test can yield false positives, triggering a litany of additional and unnecessary tests and procedures. These excess procedures may harm people and the anxiety could kill them.[23]

I reviewed the studies on the Galleri test. More may come out by the time you read this book, but based on what's out now, it's not clear if the test can do more harm than good. My conclusion was simple: Giving every American a Galleri test is a great idea, but it's not ready for prime time.

Consider the data for yourself.

In one large study, 58% of people informed by the Galleri test that they might have cancer ended up having nothing. It was also discovered that the test may miss up to 70% of cancers.[24,25] The false positive rate could be higher but, oddly, the study reported that hundreds of people "remain under review."

Further, early detection is different from prevention.[26] Simply discovering a cancer doesn't mean a life was saved. The real question is: Did the test save anyone's life? If so, did it save more lives than the lives lost from unnecessary testing in response to false positives? Many cancers discovered in the studies were already in later or incurable stages. This, as opposed to the detection of an early cancer, is what we refer to in oncology as a "turtle" — a slow-growing tumor that most people could outlive. There are also cancers that would get caught eventually before they spread, and have a favorable prognosis irrespective of when they're picked up. That may have been the case for a few of the cancers the test reportedly detected in a population of 53,744 patients who were tested in one study. Interestingly, the study did not report the stage of the cancer in about half of the people diagnosed. Why didn't the company report that information?

The company has boasted that one person was discovered to have pancreas cancer based on the test. But all we know about the case is that the same person has appeared in more than one media article. More details would be welcome. Since the Galleri test has been performed on nearly 100,000 people, one would expect numerous examples of lives saved.

The test's high false-positive rate means a lot of people get a flurry of downstream diagnostic tests and procedures, some of which have small risks. In one of the studies, the average time spent waiting and undergoing follow-up testing was 162 days.[27] Waiting for cancer test results can be hell. It can be a time of intense physiologic and mental stress. I've seen people waiting for test results prepare themselves to die. Even suicide has been reported during this anxious time. Just because follow-up tests eventually may reveal nothing doesn't mean waiting to have them can't hurt you in the meantime. The Grail-sponsored studies didn't report complications of downstream tests like colonoscopies and invasive biopsies triggered by false positives. There are also concerns about the radiation exposure of repeat imaging tests in younger people.

In reading the studies on Galleri, I saw a lot of incomplete data. The studies, which are funded by the company, do not explain why they included people with "additional risk" for cancer. They also do not report the ages of those diagnosed, whether any lives were saved, or why there is so much incomplete data.[28]

Dr. Susan Bewley, emerita professor at King's College London, called the Galleri test "ethically dubious" in the *Financial Times*. "This sort of screening test could bankrupt the [National Health Service], prioritize people who are well over those who are sick, and make people ill," Dr. Bewley said. "Screening is like a modern form of bloodletting with leeches: If you died it's because we didn't leech you early enough and if you didn't die then the leeches saved you."[29]

The company that developed the test was funded with investments from Bill Gates and Jeff Bezos. It's had some drama. It was spun out in 2016 of the DNA testing company Illumina, which became a leading Covid-testing company during the pandemic. European regulators and the U.S. Federal Trade Commission have been investigating the company following its controversial re-merger with Illumina in August 2021.[30,31]

From financial documents I learned that the chief technology officer at Illumina suddenly resigned in 2023 and dumped all his stock.[32] The chief medical officer and CEO also resigned that same year. If you are leading a company on the brink of a major cancer breakthrough revolutionizing health, one would think you'd want to keep working on it and hold on to your potentially valuable stock.

Illumina's government lobbying effort has been intense. The company hired former

UK Prime Minister David Cameron and, magically, soon after doing so, secured a contract with the UK government to fund a clinical trial. The company also added former president Barack Obama in 2022 to its Illumina Genomics Forum, where it also hosted Francis Collins, who had recently stepped down as director of the NIH, and tennis legend Chris Evert. Currently there is a massive lobbying effort to get the U.S. government to foot the bill for the test in every older American, which could cost upward of $60 billion. The effort even has a ringing endorsement from the president of the American Cancer Society's Cancer Action Network.[33] A friend of mine in Congress told me it's one of the biggest lobbying efforts he's ever seen. At the forefront of their case is the promise to close gaps in health equity.[34]

I don't mean to rain on the parade, but before we throw $60 billion in taxpayer dollars at this test, let's see how many lives it truly saves. We should also weigh the cost against other ways we could spend that large amount of money: on prenatal vitamins, buying food for hungry children in America, and ending the dumping of raw sewage into my local river.

Would I trust handing over my genetic

information to this company? Not at this point. It's not hard to imagine the mishandling of this collected genetic data. In 2023, the company mistakenly sent letters to 400 of its customers informing them they might have cancer. Half of the people had not even had the Galleri test done yet. *Yikes!* Even more concerning is that the company knew about this error but failed to disclose it until *after* its shareholder proxy vote.

I believe in early cancer detection and hope liquid biopsies can save lives in the future, but this test is not quite ready. If it is broadly rolled out now, I worry about the hundreds of thousands of people who will undergo invasive tests because of false negative results. Certainly, the medical-industrial complex is poised to generate a lot of business, but will it improve health? Before we as a medical profession and country get sold on testing all Medicare beneficiaries with a novel test, let's make sure it saves more lives than it destroys.

This is not the first time that we have been told that collecting everyone's genetic information can solve our problems. When white settlers in New Mexico and Arizona diverted water out of the Gila River, they left the Pima Indians with land they could no longer farm. To avoid starvation, the

U.S. government gave them foods similar to Spam to eat. (For younger readers, this Spam is not junk email, it's a highly processed meat that ancient people mistook as healthy.) The government food made them obese, spawning a diabetes epidemic in their nation. NIH researchers then swooped in to test their blood to look for a genetic basis for their obesity. University of Utah professor Dr. James Tabery details the obsession with a genetic cause for the manufactured epidemic.[35] "Sometimes the quest for medical knowledge gets so myopic, we can't see the forest for the trees," he told me.

Many academics and policy leaders are already suggesting that the Galleri test is an important public health campaign that can finally slash cancer deaths. I'd love that to be true, but that's an opinion. We do not have the data yet to support that belief. At the same time, we must keep an open mind. We can't be *against* the Galleri test because of the bandwagon effect we are witnessing. We must be open to the possibility that it may someday effectively detect cancers with a risk–benefit ratio that favors doing it widely.

We need better data before recommending the new liquid biopsy test for everyone. I'm not the only one who thinks so. Several UK-based genomic and computational biology scientists recently threw cold water on the Galleri parade in the *Lancet:* "The NHS can ill-afford to be a world leader in the adoption of poorly evaluated interventions that might be of little or no benefit, harm people, and waste resources that could be better used elsewhere."[36]

5. The Annual Flu Shot Runaround

Each year the medical community makes a push for everyone to get a new flu shot, the efficacy of which ranges anywhere from 5 to 60%. Vaccine makers take a gander at designing the vaccine to combat the strain expected to be dominant that year. But what if we had a universal flu shot that gave long-lasting immunity to many different flu strains, including future strains?

That's the promising work of a few scientists in the U.S. But sadly, they are struggling to get this important work done.

Using four avian influenza strains, Dr. Matthew Memoli and Dr. Jeffery Taubenberger at the NIH, have developed a universal flu vaccine that has shown incredible promise in animal studies.[37] Interestingly this vaccine is not being developed rapidly by NIH, despite it being formally proposed to the National Vaccine Advisory Committee in 2022.[38] One likely reason is that the universal flu vaccine uses traditional inactivated virus vaccine technology, not mRNA. Current enthusiasm for mRNA vaccines within the scientific community means that new vaccines that use traditional technology don't get as much funding and support.

You may be asking: If the universal flu vaccine uses traditional vaccine technology, why did it take so long to be developed? To answer this question, it's important to understand that there are many parts to an influenza virus, including the prominent H (hemagglutinin) and N (neuraminidase) parts. Hence the names H1N1, H5N1, etc.

For decades, all previous flu vaccines have been based on the assumption that they should target the H part. But Dr. Memoli's research on the N part[39] and other prior studies[40,41] have found that immunity to the N part is a better predictor of protection than the immunity to the H part. Focusing yearly vaccines on the H part may be a classic case of medical groupthink, resulting in a scientific blind spot.

Animal data with the new universal flu vaccine looks promising. It generated antibodies to many different components of the virus, including both H and the N parts as well as a cellular response involving B and T cells. It produced antibodies to a wide variety of known influenza viruses, including the 1918 influenza virus.

This promising vaccine has completed Phase 1 human trials.[42] So what is delaying the start of the next phase of human studies? The NIH and the Department of Health and Human Services have not put their full weight and funding behind it.

mRNA vaccines have been celebrated by the medical establishment as a technology that allows scientists to program in the desired protein each year to fight a virus. A universal flu shot with a non-mRNA technology is regarded by some as yesterday's junk.

A source of mine who communicated with the Gates Foundation tells me that the Foundation is not interested in further funding clinical vaccine research like Dr. Memoli's, because they are focused on mRNA vaccines.

There's also another big reason why there may not be a rush to develop this. Pharma can't make billions on it. An annual vaccine product that can be sold each flu season in perpetuity gets shareholders excited. Also, the universal flu vaccine uses naturally occurring viruses, so there isn't the precious intellectual property rights that can generate a fortune.

Sources close to the matter tell me that BARDA, the government agency that funds research, favors novel vaccine research with intellectual property rights that can pay hefty royalties back to the government.

Every year, there are stern warnings by experts of the possibility of a bird flu pandemic that could be catastrophic. It's certainly possible. But instead of top government health officials showing concern and tracking it closely, how about fast-tracking basic research and development on a promising universal flu vaccine? We don't have evidence yet that it will work in humans, but it is designed to cover H5N1 and other threatening strains of bird flu that have mortality rates as high as 50%. The recent Covid pandemic should have taught us not to take a "wait and see" approach. Influenza viruses pose a catastrophic risk to the world. We need to adopt a proactive approach to pandemic preparedness rather than just a reactive one.

And each year, as the medical establishment commands everyone to take the annual flu shot and spends billions on the crusade, it would be good to pause and consider this potential blind spot: developing a universal flu shot could save many more lives.

6. Testosterone Replacement for Men

When we doctors are asked about a new treatment, our first reaction is to find out if it's backed up by a robust study. If we don't have a study, we get uncomfortable with uncertainty. We are trained to dismiss the issue. Until recently, testosterone replacement for men has been in that gray zone. (The role of food and vitamins in overall health has also been relegated to the same medical purgatory.)

It's also easy to be turned off by all the shady pill shops pushing testosterone. But if we're being objective, we shouldn't dismiss something because we don't like those who are supporting it.

Many midlife men struggle with low energy, weight gain, sleep apnea, depressed mood, and sexual dysfunction. Sometimes they discover their free testosterone level is low upon testing and told about the option of testosterone replacement therapy (TRT).

New research is emerging about the benefits of TRT in men with low T. Doctors who frequently prescribe TRT for men tell me that they are seeing their patients feel better, increase their libido, and lose weight, which can subsequently alleviate their sleep apnea. Dr. Mark McCormick in South Florida tells me he's seen people come off their

CPAP machines with TRT. Wow. Imagine the potential implications for better health through better sleep, not to mention the savings of being off the CPAP. Poor sleep is bad for the heart and contributes to high blood pressure, weight gain, and possibly Alzheimer's.[43] Dr. McCormick is also seeing his patients on TRT exercise more and improve their self-confidence.

There are both similarities and important differences between TRT in men and hormone replacement therapy (HRT) in women. HRT and TRT work differently, and thus TRT should not be regarded as the male equivalent of HRT. Estrogen offers more profound benefits by keeping blood vessels soft and healthy in postmenopausal women. To varying degrees, both HRT and TRT result in higher bone density[44] and lower fat mass,[45] and help with blood-sugar levels in people with Type 2 diabetes.[46]

In the same way that HRT has been accused of causing breast cancer, TRT has been alleged to cause prostate cancer, an allegation that has not been well supported in studies. There are also cardiovascular concerns. TRT may increase the risk of cardiovascular problems by a small effect size in everyone who takes it, and that risk may increase when men start TRT after the onset of heart disease.

I should mention that there are known downsides of TRT. Extended use of TRT may permanently shut down the body's intrinsic production, creating a dependence on the drug after a number of years. And when a man stops taking it, he may immediately lose all the benefits it provided. It's also not easy to take. Currently it's usually taken as a cream, injection, or implantable pellets, and many men may need additional medications to prevent its side effects, such as breast swelling. Furthermore, while alleviation of sleep apnea can be dramatic with TRT, other people report the medication makes their sleep worse! TRT can also cause water retention, which is why a doctor, not a personal trainer, should evaluate a man for the therapy. Finally, TRT can cause infertility, which is why it's not recommended for men hoping to have children. There appears to be a subset of men with "low T" for whom TRT can do more harm than good. For this reason, the decision to use it should be individualized.

On the whole, after my conversations with experts in the field, it appears that many men who are ideal candidates for TRT are currently not being offered the option. It may be that modern medicine is underappreciating the value of TRT to alleviate some chronic health problems in men.

7. A Non-Debate about Children

On June 12, 2023, the U.S. Assistant Secretary for Health declared that gender-affirming care is "suicide prevention care." Trans children do indeed have an elevated suicide risk, however, no definitive study has found that surgery or puberty blockers reduce that risk, rendering the Assistant Secretary's statement an opinion rather than evidence based.

To support the claim, the Assistant Secretary cited support from the American Medical Association, the American Academy of Pediatrics, and other medical groups. But, as we've seen throughout this book, agreement among organized medicine leaders alone does not constitute evidence.

In this section, I present two prevalent views among physicians and describe the debate. The first view recognizes that on very rare occasions, some children are born with a mix of male and female anatomy. Some children assigned as boys at birth have ovaries, and some children assigned as girls at birth have male genitalia. The medical terms "intersex" and "differences in sexual development" have been used to describe these individuals, who, in this view, are the only people for whom medical intervention may be indicated.

The second view, the gender-affirming view, goes a step further. It adds that all children should pick their gender identity, even if they don't have any anatomic or genetic abnormalities. It encourages all children to pick a gender (or no gender) based on their feelings and maintains that the duty of medical professionals is to simply affirm their decision, sometimes with hormones or surgery.

In Europe, there has been a healthy debate on the topic. Academics have made arguments on each side as researchers have studied transgender children who have been treated over time. In the UK, the National Health Service commissioned a formal review of the research on the topic and concluded that puberty blockers were not supported by good evidence and that they have not been shown to be safe and effective. As a result of this formal review of the literature, in 2024 the UK banned puberty blockers except in clinical trials. The review cited a study showing that 71% of children who took puberty blockers had no improvement in their mental health and about one third did worse.[47] A similar trend has been observed in other European countries. In 2022, Sweden updated their guidelines to further restrict children from accessing gender-affirming care, stating that the evidence for "hormonal interventions" for minors is "of low quality" and that treatments may present risks.[48] And most recently, a 2024 Danish study found that the suicide risk in transgender children was driven by the high rate and severity of their underlying mental health disorders, not by their gender identity.[49] In other words, hormones and transition surgery may have no impact on lowering suicide risk. That's the conversation among doctors in Europe.

In the U.S., the debate is much different. Some experts are afraid to speak up. The story of Brown University's Dr. Lisa Littman illustrates why.

Dr. Littman gathered data from surveys of hundreds of parents of transgender children and identified common characteristics. She described how cases of youth identifying as transgender occurred in clusters rather than randomly in the population, and many had underlying mental health disorders.[50] She found that the clusters often included girls who binged on social media. Some physicians have speculated that girls may be particularly vulnerable to images — a trend seen in anorexia, which also affects girls far more than boys.

Littman's findings challenged the gender-affirming view, including the position of some powerful academic leaders. Although the study was small, it suggested that if transgenderism was biologic, one would expect a more random distribution in the population, not a social contagion among clusters of girls bingeing on social media. The medical journal that published her study was intensely pressured to retract it. The journal ultimately forced Dr. Littman to go back and make several minor changes after it was published, the most emblematic of which was watering down the title, from "Rapid-Onset Gender Dysphoria in Adolescents and Young Adults: A Study of Parental Reports" to "Parent Reports of Adolescents and Young Adults Perceived to Show Signs of a Rapid Onset of Gender Dysphoria." But not a single data point was changed. Forcing her to change her words was a modern-day tarring and feathering. Critics suddenly suggested the article was corrected, as if it had contained data errors — which it hadn't.

For the record, it's unheard of for a journal to force a researcher to change the title of their research study after it's published.

Brown University jumped into the issue and smacked her down. The institution distanced itself from her and the study, and did not renew her contract, despite her meeting all performance benchmarks. The university openly criticized the study in its statement, saying that "the conclusions of the study could be used to discredit efforts to support transgender youth." Later in the same long press release, the university affirmed its commitment to academic freedom and boasted that it was "proud to be among the first universities to include medical care for gender reassignment."[51] The medical establishment put Dr. Littman through hell. What was her crime? She published a study with results that some people didn't like.

There was no open debate about the data. Similarly, in 2021, American Academy of Pediatrics (AAP) member Dr. Julia Mason submitted a resolution within the organization suggesting that it hold off on promoting transition surgery for minors until research demonstrated long-term safety and patient benefits. The resolution generated a lot of engagement, with 80% of committee input favoring presenting the resolution to their Annual Leadership Forum. But oddly, the resolution never left the committee. It was not advanced for consideration by senior leadership. Dr. Mason later commented that many of the associations that recommend gender-affirming care were doing so because "it's the position of a few activists that have captured key committees at medical societies."[52]

A past president of the AAP, Dr. Joseph Zanga, argued that the AAP has been unwilling to discuss the appropriateness of medical intervention for transgender youth. He said, "The science says that children and adolescents are not capable of making these kinds of decisions." But the topic of affirming gender with hormones and surgery was not debated at AAP conferences. Instead, AAP members discussed topics like promoting recycling. When Dr. Zanga submitted a dissenting commentary questioning gender-affirming care for publication in his AAP state chapter newsletter, it was rejected.

Mayo Clinic's former associate dean for research, Dr. Michael Joyner, is an accomplished and oft-cited expert in exercise physiology. Shortly after stating his opinion to the *New York Times* that athletes who have gone through male puberty may have an unfair advantage competing against women, Mayo suspended him and cut his pay.[53] In a letter they sent to him, Mayo told him he had "failed to communicate in accordance with prescribed messaging."[54] Dr. Joyner had not plagiarized research or committed a mistake that killed a patient (both of which, by the way, are not fireable offenses at many medical centers).

He did something far worse: Dr. Joyner voiced an opinion different from that of his medical school's administration.

Dr. Miriam Grossman, a child psychiatrist who had a long career at UCLA, describes the collective opinion of organized medicine as "the Castro Consensus" in her book *Lost in Trans Nation.*[55] She's referring to a time when Cuba's former president Fidel Castro removed other candidates from the ballot, then announced his referendum to be a national consensus. Regardless of which view you hold on this issue, we should all agree that the present debate is not going well.

Should both sides of a scientific controversy be discussed? Laura Helmuth, editor in chief of one of the most prestigious scientific journals, *Scientific American,* recently argued no. She issued a statement in 2023, providing a list of scientific topics that she said "we don't need to be both-sidesing" or asking questions about.[56] The list included gender-affirming care for trans people, vaccines, and other topics. I wonder what she would say about the rotavirus or anthrax vaccines? After dangerous risks emerged, both vaccines were pulled off the market after they were strongly recommended or required.

The trans topic understandably arouses high emotions given the gravitas of adults making decisions about a vulnerable population. What's clear is that when parents are told that they must consent to hormones or surgery for their child in order to prevent suicide, the recommendation is not based on evidence even when it is presented as evidence-based. In addition, parents are told that puberty blockers have no long-term complications — a claim challenged by a 2024 study suggesting that some of their effects may not be reversible.[57] In a bid to best nurture and care for our children, we need robust research and an open forum of scientific ideas.

8. Tongue-Tied America

Increasingly, lactation consultants, dentists, and pediatricians are recommending cutting the base of the tongue of infants for a condition called "tongue-tie." This is meant to help with suckling and breast-feeding. The procedure is done by holding open the baby's mouth and snipping the frenulum under the tongue. While some tongue-tied babies appear to breastfeed better after the procedure, some may not — due to the pain.

There's not good evidence to support the procedure. It's another widespread practice that needs a robust clinical trial before babies are routinely subjected to the procedure. The best data we have is from a 2017 Cochrane review, which failed to find a positive benefit on breast-feeding outcomes.[58]

Some dentists and physicians have made dubious claims that the procedure can help a child's speech or reduce sleep apnea later in life — claims lacking any scientific support. In fact, I wonder if tongue-cutting could have the opposite effect.

Regardless, it's now a new cottage industry in America, with some dentists performing over a hundred per week, according to the *New York Times*.[59] What's more concerning is that some clinicians are also cutting a baby's cheeks where they join with the side of the tongue. I sought out good data on that but couldn't find any.

Yet another procedure commonly done at the same time as cutting the cheeks and tongue is cutting the inside of the upper lip. For this one, the American Academy of Otolaryngology–Head and Neck Surgery recently denounced it as a procedure that "should not be performed."[60]

My colleagues and I have seen an alarming overuse of lip cutting by some dentists and physicians treating children of low-income families. Medicaid billing records submitted to our Global Appropriateness Measures consortium[61] show that cutting the mouths of children is the dominant procedure performed by some dentists. Perhaps the criteria used by these physicians is so broad that if the baby does not appear to perfectly extend its tongue, it gets labeled as tongue-tied, strapped down, and sliced in four spots of its mouth.

I asked an ENT colleague I trust about this, and he told me that a fraction of select kids may benefit from the tongue release, but the procedure is applied far too indiscriminately.

Before we cut the mouths of millions of children, we should study if it's helping with the intended benefits and whether or not the procedure has any long-term consequences. If it does help some children, let's identify the characteristics of kids who benefit most, so parents can make an informed decision.

The truth of whether tongue, lip, or cheek cutting helps or hurts children can be answered definitively with a proper clinical trial. But who's going to fund such a study?

The NIH? Highly unlikely. Pharma? No way. The AAP? Slim chance. A community of infants? Don't count on it. Tragically, many medical controversies like this can be settled, but instead lingers in a scientific vacuum backfilled with opinions. We cannot continue to allow major clinical questions to live in the Bermuda Triangle of no funding. The void of data on mouth cutting procedures embodies a major problem in our $4.5 trillion health care system in the U.S.: Answering important clinical questions is rarely on anyone's funding radar.

The saga of the AAP getting peanut allergy prevention wrong for 15 years carries an important lesson: If there is uncertainty about a practice or a controversy in the field, do a proper study *before* the practice becomes widely adopted.

9. GLP-1 Drugs Save Lives

Highly celebrated GLP-1 medications like Ozempic and Rybelsus appear to be effective not only for losing weight, but also in reducing the health problems associated with obesity such as heart disease, liver disease, and renal failure. But studies showing these benefits have looked at outcomes in the first few years of use. In the long run, are these medications good for your health? While we can have our opinions, the truth is we don't yet know.

This class of medications appears to both reduce excess fat *and* muscle mass. Muscle mass is the leading predictor of longevity. Loss of muscle mass is a component of the frailty syndrome.[62] And loss of muscle mass is one reason why doctors who prescribe GLP-1 drugs are keen to make sure that people taking them exercise and get enough protein in their diet.

While it appears that we are seeing exciting health benefits from these medications, we have to be open to the fact that future research could tell us that people on them long-term ultimately live longer, or shorter lives.

10. Mammograms for Low-Risk Women

If you ask experts, "How do we fix health care?" some will promptly respond: more prevention. Follow up on that standard answer, and often people claim we need to increase mammogram rates. It's hard to oppose mammograms, because who doesn't want to protect women from breast cancer? But you might be surprised to know that the data supporting the most recent broadening of mammogram recommendations are strikingly flimsy.

In 2023, the U.S. Preventive Services

Task Force lowered the recommended age for low-risk women to start getting mammograms from 50 to 40 years of age. You would think that recommending that millions of healthy, low-risk women in their 40s should receive an uncomfortable medical procedure with radiation exposure would be supported by clinical trials showing that it saves lives. But that wasn't the case. There was not a single clinical trial demonstrating that mammograms in low-risk women in their forties saves lives.[63]

Supporters of the new recommendation might argue that it's so obvious that we don't need a good study. After all, they may have once seen a 40-year-old woman get diagnosed with early breast cancer via a mammogram. But that's not how science works. Maybe that cancer was a "turtle." And false positives are common. About half of women who get an annual mammogram will experience a false positive over a ten-year period, according to the American Cancer Society. That may lead to unnecessary surgical procedures and additional radiation exposures — not to mention the stress of being told you might have cancer.[64]

Does mass mammography screening in low-risk women in their forties save lives? The question has yet to be answered.

Some advocates of the new recommendation believe we don't need to do proper clinical trials because they "know" it saves lives. That's a dangerous way of thinking. Sure, it's fine to have opinions based on one's bedside observations, but issuing major health recommendations based on opinion alone is exactly how we've seen so many errors occur in modern medicine. Also, the everyone-needs-to-do-this-because-we-say-so mentality is medical paternalism — an attitude that has severely damaged the public trust in recent decades.

We should not cut corners on science. That means we can make a recommendation, such as encouraging all women in their forties to get a mammogram, as long as we tell women this advice is based on an opinion rather than studies showing the procedure saves lives. Once a study is conducted and the results are in, we must be open to evolving our position, whether or not it supports conventional thinking.

PARACHUTES

As above with mammograms, sometimes people make an argument that there's no need to do a randomized trial to study a medical intervention "because it's so obvious" and "we just know it to be true."

The argument that there's no need to do a proper study is what I call the parachute argument. In 2003, two authors in the medical journal *BMJ* explained how there was no need for a randomized trial to establish that parachutes save lives.[65] Randomized trials divide participants into groups that receive the intervention and those that do not, so researchers can gauge the effect of the intervention. The authors are right: It would be unethical to ask half of a study population to jump out of an airplane without a parachute to confirm that the device saves lives. Everyone agrees we can learn from deductive reasoning and observational experience.

However, the randomized trial model is not the only way to gain scientific knowledge. And the we-don't-need-a-trial argument is selectively applied. If someone wants to push a medical intervention into the mainstream, they argue we don't need a clinical trial: It's a parachute! Conversely, if they don't like a common-sense idea, they might say we can't embrace it unless we have a randomized trial.

Sadly today, the parachute argument is being weaponized to dismiss the call to study certain health recommendations. During the recent pandemic, zealots on both sides used the we-don't-need-a study-because-we-know-it-works argument to justify their positions. Again, it was the parachute argument.

The pandemic was not a one-off in how the medical establishment works. In fact, it was more the norm than the exception. For example, decades have passed in which heart stents were used to "open up" blocked arteries in the heart. Why study that? It's obvious the procedure was doing good — or so we thought.

After hundreds of thousands of heart stents were put into people's bodies (at a high price tag), the aptly named COURAGE trial[66] revealed that heart stents have zero impact on prolonging one's life, unless the stent is placed during an active heart attack. Stents can alleviate angina (chronic chest discomfort) symptoms, but they don't extend patients' lives.

But stents had been considered parachutes. We saw blockages pushed open right in front of our eyes, people argued. And then we learned that stents disrupt the lining of the inside of the blood vessel and can *cause* a blockage — a phenomenon known as in-stent thrombosis. The percentage of people treated with a heart stent today is way down from the days before the COURAGE trial.

We can use clinical wisdom to recommend

interventions, but the medical establishment owes it to the public to do clinical trials before making sweeping recommendations for the masses. We can do both: make recommendations based on opinion while insisting on proper studies to inform big recommendations.

Declaring that desirable interventions are parachutes is intellectually lazy and a dishonest way to do public-health policy. Ultimately, the data catch up and trust in the profession is eroded. Now, more than ever, the public is hungry for honesty and humility.

The Father of Evidence-Based Medicine: Temporarily Suspend Your Biases

Many of the interventions presented in this chapter — the use of fluoride, liquid biopsies, and mammograms for women in their forties — have to do with prevention. To further explore this topic, let's look at the teachings of Dr. David Sackett, the late Oxford and McMaster professor who's known as the father of evidence-based medicine.

Dr. Sackett warned that preventive medicine had become arrogant, aggressively assertive, and presumptuous. The medical profession, he explained, was pushing preventive interventions that had not yet been proven with proper studies. Dr. Sackett said that numerous broadly recommended preventive interventions in healthy people had been disastrous, and that studies of them found they did more harm than good. Among many examples, he cited the reckless American Academy of Pediatrics recommendation to have babies sleep on their stomach — later reversed when people learned sleeping face down *increased* rates of sudden death.

Dr. Sackett lambasted people and institutions who dole out unscientific guidelines. The "experts" are to blame for allowing their own gain or a "narcissistic need for public acclaim" to lead them to advocate preventive practices that haven't been validated in rigorous studies, Sackett said.[67] "Not only do they abuse their positions by advocating unproven 'preventives,' they also stifle dissent," he said.

Such experts refuse to learn from history until they make it themselves, Dr. Sackett said.

Toward the end of his career, he coauthored an article in the *BMJ* stating that evidence-based medicine is not a cookbook. Instead, it requires careful judgment. "Good doctors use both individual clinical expertise and the best available external evidence, and neither alone is enough," he wrote.[68]

Asking Questions

In science, you have to be able to ask questions. So let me pose a big one: Could it be that many of our modern-day health crises were caused by (or hastened by) the hubris of the medical establishment?

Experts told people *for decades* that opioids were not addictive — igniting the opioid crisis. They insisted infants avoid peanut butter — fueling the peanut allergy epidemic. They demonized natural fat in foods — driving people to processed carbohydrates as obesity rates soared. They prescribed antibiotics haphazardly — altering the gut microbiomes of a generation and causing a drug-resistant bacteria epidemic. They unfairly used fear to scare women away from HRT, resulting in a generation of women being denied the life-extending and quality of life benefits. And some might say that "experts" experimented on a bat coronavirus in the lab for no good reason, causing a global pandemic.

Medical dogma continues to loom large. Sometimes because people are railroaded for asking questions, and sometimes because loud medical establishment leaders who got things perfectly backward have never apologized for their decades-long hubris.

The question of whether many of our current health crises are man-made rears its head up everyday in the hospital and at my research team meeting where we track the most urgent issues in our $4.5 trillion health care ecosystem.

Asking questions has become forbidden in some circles. But asking questions is not the problem, it's the solution.

Looking Ahead

When medicine makes recommendations based on sound studies, our profession shines. We do a lot of good and reduce the burden of harm on a population. But when we make recommendations based on opinion, we do not have a great track record.

We must hold high the scientific method and recognize our biases. As Dr. Festinger pointed out, we all have a natural tendency to dismiss information we simply don't like. Calling an intervention a "parachute" when it deserves a proper study is one way smart people make bad policy.

Second, sometimes in medicine, the right answer is "I don't know." As we saw with the peanut abstinence recommendation, there was a feeling among medical leaders that they needed to tell people *something* — even though they didn't know what. "We don't know" may be our best answer. The public can be forgiving if we are honest.

Third, health professionals and the public must know which recommendations are based on opinion and which are based on robust medical evidence. Opinion-based recommendations should never be presented as evidence-based.

Fourth, the best way to fight bad ideas is with better ideas, not by canceling scientists. The open forum of scientific debate is becoming increasingly intolerant. When Barack Obama ran for president, he was asked what his favorite book was. He cited *Team of Rivals,* a book about President Abraham Lincoln's practice of surrounding himself with cabinet members who disagreed with him and challenged him. All leaders — in medicine and other industries — should consider the value of this type of immersion in competing ideas.

Finally, scientists and business innovators in medicine alike should be inspired to think differently and challenge deeply held assumptions in the field. Americans are getting sicker as health care's stakeholders are getting richer. We need to listen to the young students, nurses, and doctors who are proposing bold new ways to deliver care today.

The era of medical dogma is far from over. If we asked the right questions about current medical practices and did the proper scientific study to answer them, the results would rock our world.

In an era of increased connectedness, the sway of groupthink may be magnified. All the more reason why we must consciously maintain our objectivity in everything we do. That includes learning from people we don't like who say things we don't like.

French physician Dr. Claude Bernard, who lived from 1813 to 1878, is considered to be the founder of modern medicine.[69] He wrote a lot about bias. He asserted that we all have our biases; we cannot eliminate them. Instead, we need to recognize them and *actively* suspend them as best we can during an experiment. He urged scientists to enter into a hyper-skeptical state of being while gathering new information. It requires effort, he argued. Dr. Bernard maintained that we can't erase our biases, but being our own antagonist makes our experiments better. That was back in the 1800s, but his words were prophetic.

If Dr. Bernard were alive today, he would implore all of us to be open-minded when new information challenges our deeply held beliefs. When we are, everyone thrives. This is true in medicine as well as in other areas of our lives.

ACKNOWLEDGMENTS

I'm very grateful to Marshall Allen, who was the senior editor of the book. Marshall brought his wisdom and experience as one of the nation's leading health-care investigative journalists to the project in the form of mentorship and editorial guidance. Thank you to Nancy Miller at Bloomsbury for believing so strongly in this book and for your editorial genius as well. I'd also like to express my appreciation to Mansur Shaheen, Paul Attia, Asonganyi Aminkeng, Andrea Michele Mackenzie, and Faith Magwenzi for their excellent ideas; and to Christi Walsh for keeping both my practice and my research projects running smoothly. Thank you to Dr. Jeremy Greene for your command of medical history; Leslie Hansen Lindner, Sina Haeri (Ouma), Amanda Nickles Fader, Barbara Levy (Visana), and Dan Martin for your clinical and obstetrical wisdom; and Gary Taubes and Orrin Devinsky for your knowledge of the history of saturated fat. Thanks to Peter and Jill Attia for our conversations about life, friendship, health, and longevity; and Dr. Jeff Kerr, David Goldhill, and Leah Binder for your big ideas. Thank you to Dr. John Alverdy from the University of Chicago, Dr. Edwin Kim from the University of North Carolina, and the almighty Malina Manger for allowing me to write this book by keeping my life efficient and seamless. Thanks to Alexander for mowing the lawn and to Nora for your big hugs. Special thanks to Dr. Vinay Prasad (the great sensei), Tracy Beth Høeg, Dr. Adam Cifu, Dr. John Mandrola, and Dr. Zubin Damania. You inspire me and I learn from all of you.

NOTES

Chapter 1: The Salem Peanut Trial

1. S. H. Sicherer et al., "Prevalence of Peanut and Tree Nut Allergy in the U.S. Determined by a Random Digit Dial Telephone Survey," *Journal of Allergy and Clinical Immunology* 103, no. 4 (April 1999): 559–62, doi:10.1016/s0091-6749(99)70224-1, PMID:10200001.
2. R. S. Gupta et al., "The Public Health Impact of Parent-Reported Childhood Food Allergies in the United States," *Pediatrics* 142, no. 6 (2018), doi:10.1542/peds.2018-1235.
3. M. Jackson, *Allergy: The History of a Modern Malady* (London: Reaktion Books, 2006).
4. American Academy of Pediatrics Committee on Nutrition, "Hypoallergenic Infant Formulas," *Pediatrics* 106, no. 2 (August 2000):

346–49, doi:10.1542/peds.106.2.346.

5. Committee on Toxicity of Chemicals in Food, Consumer Products and the Environment, *Peanut Allergy* (London: UK Department of Health, 1998).
6. J. O. Hourihane, T. P. Dean, and J. O. Warner, "Peanut Allergy in Relation to Heredity, Maternal Diet, and Other Atopic Diseases: Results of a Questionnaire Survey, Skin Prick Testing, and Food Challenges," *BMJ: British Medical Journal* 313, no. 7056 (August 31, 1996): 518–21.
7. S. V. Lynch et al., "Effects of Early-Life Exposure to Allergens and Bacteria on Recurrent Wheeze and Atopy in Urban Children," *Journal of Allergy and Clinical Immunology* 134, no. 3 (September 2014): 593–601.
8. D. E. Fox and G. Lack., "Peanut Allergy," *Lancet* 352, no. 9129 (August 29, 1998): 741.
9. G. Du Toit et al., "Early Consumption of Peanuts in Infancy Is Associated with a Low Prevalence of Peanut Allergy," *Journal of Allergy and Clinical Immunology* 122, no. 5 (2008): 984–91.
10. M. S. Motosue et al., "National Trends in Emergency Department Visits and Hospitalizations for Food-Induced

Anaphylaxis in U.S. Children," *Pediatric Allergy and Immunology* 29 (2018): 538–44.

11. "The Prevalence of Peanut Allergy Has Trebled in 15 Years," *Economist,* October 3, 2019.
12. D. Scott, "Can We Solve the EpiPen Cost Crisis?" *Vox,* April 4, 2023, https://www.vox.com/policy/23658275/epipen-cost-price-how-much.
13. G. Du Toit et al., "Randomized Trial of Peanut Consumption in Infants at Risk for Peanut Allergy," *New England Journal of Medicine* 372 (2015): 803–13.
14. S. H. Sicherer, "New Guidelines Detail Use of 'Infant-Safe' Peanut to Prevent Allergy," *AAP News,* January 5, 2017.
15. A. Togias et al., "Addendum Guidelines for the Prevention of Peanut Allergy in the United States: Report of the National Institute of Allergy and Infectious Diseases-Sponsored Expert Panel," *Journal of Pediatric Nursing* 32 (January–February 2017): 91–98.
16. E. Donnelly, "Mom Shamed for Letting Her Kid Eat a Peanut Butter Sandwich While Shopping at Target," Yahoo Life, April 12, 2018, https://www.yahoo.com/lifestyle/mom-shamed-letting-kid-eat-peanut-butter-sandwich

-shopping-target-really-awful-105216945.html.

17. American Academy of Pediatrics, full text of "Full Filing" for fiscal year ending June 2022, ProPublica Nonprofit Explorer, accessed April 8, 2024, https://projects.propublica.org/nonprofits/organizations/362275597/202310889349300016/full.
18. G. Du Toit et al. and the Immune Tolerance Network LEAP-Trio Trial Team, "Follow-Up to Adolescence after Early Peanut Introduction for Allergy Prevention," *NEJM Evidence* 3, no. 6 (June 2024), doi:10.1056/EVIDoa2300311.
19. U.S. Food and Drug Administration, "FDA Approves First Medication to Help Reduce Allergic Reactions to Multiple Foods after Accidental Exposure," press release, February 16, 2024.

Chapter 2: OMG HRT

1. E. Barrett-Connor and T. L. Bush, "Estrogen and Coronary Heart Disease in Women," *Journal of the American Medical Association* 265, no. 14 (April 10, 1991).
2. A. Bluming and C. Tavris, *Estrogen*

Matters (New York: Little, Brown Spark, 2018).

3. National Heart, Lung, and Blood Institute, "NHLBI Stops Trial of Estrogen Plus Progestin Due to Increased Breast Cancer Risk, Lack of Overall Benefit," National Institutes of Health, news release, July 9, 2002.
4. Personal communication with Dr. R. Langer, December 1, 2023.
5. R. D. Langer, "The Evidence Base for HRT: What Can We Believe?" *Climacteric* 20, no. 2 (2017): 91–96, doi:10.1080/13697137.2017.1280251.
6. A. Z. Bluming, H. N. Hodis, and R. D. Langer, " 'Tis But a Scratch: A Critical Review of the Women's Health Initiative Evidence Associating Menopausal Hormone Therapy with the Risk of Breast Cancer," *Menopause* 30, no. 12 (December 1, 2023): 1241–45.
7. J. E. Rossouw, "Estrogens for Prevention of Coronary Heart Disease: Putting the Brakes on the Bandwagon," *Circulation* 94 (December 1996): 2982–85.
8. This is according to a transcript of the lecture, which had been recorded by Dr. A. Bluming.

9. Quoted in Bluming and Tavris, *Estrogen Matters*.
10. Personal communication with Dr. J. Manson, January 11, 2024.
11. J. H. Wuest et al., "The Degree of Coronary Atherosclerosis in Bilaterally Oophorectomized Women," *Circulation* 7 (1953): 801–9.
12. "Eight Strange and Wonderful Facts About Octopuses," Shedd Aquarium, September 6, 2023, https://www.sheddaquarium.org/stories/eight-strange-and-wonderful-facts-about-octopuses.
13. S. R. Salpeter et al., "Mortality Associated with Hormone Replacement Therapy in Younger and Older Women," *Journal of General Internal Medicine* 19 (2004): 791–804.
14. Bluming and Tavris, *Estrogen Matters*.
15. M. S. Christianson et al., "Menopause Education: Needs Assessment of American Obstetrics and Gynecology Residents," *Menopause* 20, no. 11 (November 2013): 1120–25.
16. L. Facher, "AAMC, the Medical School Trade Association, Gave $500,000 To Dark Money Group In 2018," Stat, August 11, 2020, https://www.statnews.com/2020/08/11

/aamc-citizens-truth-drug-pricing/.
17. A. Paganini-Hill and V. W. Henderson, "Estrogen Replacement Therapy and Risk of Alzheimer Disease," *Archives of Internal Medicine* (October 28, 1996).
18. W. A. Rocca et al., "Long-Term Effects of Bilateral Oophorectomy on Brain Aging: Unanswered Questions from the Mayo Clinic Cohort Study of Oophorectomy and Aging," *Women's Health* (London) 5, no. 1 (January 2009): 39–48.
19. J. W. Simpkins et al., "Role of Estrogen Replacement Therapy in Memory Enhancement and the Prevention of Neuronal Loss Associated with Alzheimer's Disease," *American Journal of Medicine* 103, no. 3, supp. 1 (September 22, 1997): S19–25.
20. R. N. Saleh et al., "Hormone Replacement Therapy Is Associated with Improved Cognition and Larger Brain Volumes in At-Risk *APOE4* Women: Results from the European Prevention of Alzheimer's Disease (EPAD) Cohort," *Alzheimer's Research and Therapy* 15, no. 1 (January 9, 2023): 10.
21. Y. Z. Bagger et al., "Early Postmenopausal Hormone Therapy

May Prevent Cognitive Impairment Later in Life," *Menopause* 12, no. 1 (January–February 2005): 12–17.
22. C. H. van Dyck et al., "Lecanemab in Early Alzheimer's Disease," *New England Journal of Medicine* 388 (2023): 9–21.
23. P. Belluck, "New Federal Decisions Make Alzheimer's Drug Leqembi Widely Accessible," *New York Times*, July 6, 2023.
24. C. Downey, M. Kelly, and J. F. Quinlan, "Changing Trends in the Mortality Rate at 1-year Post Hip Fracture: A Systematic Review," *World Journal of Orthopedics* 10, no. 3 (March 18, 2019): 166–75.
25. N. S. Weiss et al., "Decreased Risk of Fractures of the Hip and Lower Forearm with Postmenopausal Use of Estrogen," *New England Journal of Medicine* 303, no. 21 (November 20, 1980): 1195–98.
26. D. P. Kiel et al., "Hip Fracture and the Use of Estrogens in Postmenopausal Women: The Framingham Study," *New England Journal of Medicine* 317, no. 19 (November 5, 1987): 1169–74.
27. J. F. Wilson, "New Treatments for Growing Scourge of Brittle Bones,"

Annals of Internal Medicine 140, no. 2 (January 20, 2004): 153–56, doi:10.7326/0003-4819-140-2-200401200-00037, PMID:14734352.

28. "Osteoporosis," *Journal of the American Medical Association* 252, no. 6 (1984): 799–802.
29. Barrett-Connor and Bush, "Estrogen and Coronary Heart Disease in Women."
30. J. Corliss, "One in Five People at Hisk of Heart Disease Shuns Statins," *Harvard Health Letter,* June 1, 2023, https://www.health.harvard.edu/heart-health/one-in-five-people-at-risk-of-heart-disease-shuns-statins.
31. F. Grodstein et al., "A Prospective, Observational Study of Postmenopausal Hormone Therapy and Primary Prevention of Cardiovascular Disease," *Annals of Internal Medicine* 133, no. 12 (December 19, 2000): 933–41.
32. T. S. Mikkola et al., "Increased Cardiovascular Mortality Risk in Women Discontinuing Postmenopausal Hormone Therapy," *Journal of Clinical Endocrinology and Metabolism* 100, no. 12 (December 2015): 4588–94.
33. L. L. Schierbeck et al., "Effect of Hormone Replacement Therapy on

Cardiovascular Events in Recently Postmenopausal Women: Randomised Trial," *BMJ: British Medical Journal* 345 (October 9, 2012).
34. H. M. P. Boardman et al., "Hormone Therapy for Preventing Cardiovascular Disease in Both Healthy Post-Menopausal Women and Post-Menopausal Women with Pre-Existing Cardiovascular Disease," *Cochrane Database of Systematic Reviews,* no. 3 (2015), doi:10.1002/14651858.CD002229.pub4.
35. J. R. Johnson et al., "Menopausal Hormone Therapy and Risk of Colorectal Cancer," *Cancer Epidemiology, Biomarkers and Prevention* 18, no. 1 (January 2009): 196–203.
36. J. S. Hildebrand et al., "Colorectal Cancer Incidence and Postmenopausal Hormone Use by Type, Recency, and Duration in Cancer Prevention Study II," *Cancer Epidemiology, Biomarkers and Prevention* 18, no. 11 (November 2009): 2835–41.
37. G. Rennert et al., "Use of Hormone Replacement Therapy and the Risk of Colorectal Cancer," *Journal of Clinical Oncology* 27, no. 27 (September 2009): 4542–47.

38. K. L. Margolis et al., "Effect of Oestrogen Plus Progestin on the Incidence of Diabetes in Postmenopausal Women: Results from the Women's Health Initiative Hormone Trial," *Diabetologia* 47, no. 17 (July 2004): 1175–87.
39. J. E. Manson et al., "The Women's Health Initiative Hormone Therapy Trials: Update and Overview of Health Outcomes During the Intervention and Post-Stopping Phases," *Journal of the American Medical Association* 310, no 13. (October 2, 2013): 1353–68.
40. F. Mauvais-Jarvis et al., "Menopausal Hormone Therapy and Type 2 Diabetes Prevention: Evidence, Mechanisms, and Clinical Implications," *Endocrine Reviews* 38, no. 3 (June 1, 2017): 173–88.
41. National Institute of Diabetes and Digestive and Kidney Diseases, "Obesity and Overweight Statistics," accessed January 26, 2024, https://www.niddk.nih.gov/health-information/health-statistics/overweight-obesity.
42. Centers for Disease Control and Prevention, *National Diabetes Statistics Report: Estimates of Diabetes and Its Burden in the United States,* 2023,

https://www.cdc.gov/diabetes/data/statistics-report/index.html.

43. J. Passos-Soares et al., "Association Between Osteoporosis Treatment and Severe Periodontitis in Postmenopausal Women," *Menopause* 24, no. 7 (July 2017): 789–95.
44. K. Y. Park et al., "Association of Periodontitis with Menopause and Hormone Replacement Therapy: A Hospital Cohort Study Using a Common Data Model," *Journal of Periodontal and Implant Science* 53, no. 3 (June 2023): 184–93.
45. H. Golman, "FDA Approves First Drug Designed to Treat Hot Flashes," *Harvard Health Letter,* August 1, 2023, https://www.health.harvard.edu/womens-health/fda-approves-first-drug-designed-to-treat-hot-flashes.
46. Information on the Advancing Health After Hysterectomy Foundation is available at MenopauseLearning.com.
47. P. M. Sarrel et al., "The Mortality Toll of Estrogen Avoidance: An Analysis of Excess Deaths Among Hysterectomized Women Aged 50 to 59 Years," *American Journal of Public Health* 103, no. 9 (September 2013): 1583–88.

48. R. D. Langer et al., "Menopausal Hormone Therapy for Primary Prevention: Why the USPSTF Is Wrong," *Climacteric* 20, no. 5 (2017): 402–13.
49. B. Levy and J. Simon, "A Contemporary View of Menopausal Hormone Therapy," *Obstetrics and Gynecology* (2024), doi:10.1097/AOG.0000000000005553.
50. B. Ehrenreich, "The 2006 *Time* 100: Scientists & Thinkers: Jacques Rossouw," *Time,* May 8, 2006.
51. Listed in the NIH staff directory and on the NIH website as of December 1, 2023.
52. "Best Medicine Scientists," Research.com, accessed February 13, 2024, https://research.com/scientists-rankings/medicine.
53. J. E. Manson and A. M. Kaunitz, "Menopause Management: Getting Clinical Care Back on Track," *New England Journal of Medicine* 374, no. 9 (March 3, 2016): 803–6.
54. P. Attia, "#253 — Hormone replacement therapy and the Women's Health Initiative: re-examining the results, the link to breast cancer, and weighing the risk vs reward of HRT | JoAnn Manson, M.D.," in

The Peter Attia Drive (podcast), May 8, 2023, https://peterattiamd.com/joannmanson/.

55. C. Thomson and G. Anderson, for the WHI Steering Committee, "RE: Women Have Been Misled about Menopause," *New York Times,* February 26, 2023.

Chapter 3: "No Downsides to Antibiotics"

1. "The Microbiome," The Nutrition Source, Harvard T. H. Chan School of Public Health, accessed February 3, 2024, https://www.hsph.harvard.edu/nutritionsource/microbiome.
2. Centers for Disease Control and Prevention, "Measuring Outpatient Antibiotic Prescribing: Appropriateness of Outpatient Antibiotic Prescribing," accessed December 21, 2023, https://www.cdc.gov/antibiotic-use/data/outpatient-prescribing/index.html.
3. P. D. Tamma et al., "Association of Adverse Events with Antibiotic Use in Hospitalized Patients," *JAMA Internal Medicine* 177, no. 9 (2017): 1308–15.
4. T. Yatsunenko et al., "Human Gut Microbiome Viewed Across Age and Geography," *Nature* 486 (2012): 222–27.

5. L. M. Cox and M. J. Blaser, "Antibiotics in Early Life and Obesity," *Nature Reviews Endocrinology* 11, no. 3 (March 2015): 182–90.
6. I. Cho et al., "Antibiotics in Early Life Alter the Murine Colonic Microbiome and Adiposity," *Nature* 488 (2012): 621–26.
7. L. Cox et al., "Microbiota Primed for Obesity," *Cell* 158, no. 4 (August 14, 2014): 705–21.
8. A. Aversa et al., "Association of Infant Antibiotic Exposure with Childhood Health Outcomes," *Mayo Clinic Proceedings* 96, no. 1 (2021): 66–77.
9. M. A. Beier et al., "Early Life Antibiotic Exposure and Incident Chronic Diseases in Childhood" (oral presentation, International Conference on Pharmacoepidemiology and Therapeutic Risk Management, August 23–25, 2021).
10. K. S. Bongers et al., "Antibiotics Cause Metabolic Changes in Mice Primarily through Microbiome Modulation Rather than Behavioral Changes," *PLOS One* 17, no. 3 (March 17, 2022), doi:10.1371/journal.pone.0265023.
11. A. F. Schulfer et al., "Intergenerational Transfer of Antibiotic-Perturbed

Microbiota Enhances Colitis in Susceptible Mice," *Nature Microbiology* 3, no. 2 (February 2018): 234–42.

12. H. S. Yoon et al., "*Akkermansia muciniphila* Secretes a Glucagon-Like Peptide-1-Inducing Protein that Improves Glucose Homeostasis and Ameliorates Metabolic Disease in Mice," *Nature Microbiology* 6, no. 5 (May 2021): 563–73.
13. F. Perraudeau et al., "Improvements to Postprandial Glucose Control in Subjects with Type 2 Diabetes: A Multicenter, Double Blind, Randomized Placebo-Controlled Trial of a Novel Probiotic Formulation," *BMJ Open Diabetes Research and Care* 8, no. 1 (2020), doi:10.1136/bmjdrc-2020-001319.
14. L. N. Segal and M. J. Blaser, "A Brave New World: The Lung Microbiota in an Era of Change," *Annals of the American Thoracic Society* 11, supp. 1 (January 2014): S21–27.
15. SCImago Journal and Country Rank, 2024, https://www.scimagojr.com/journalrank.php?category=2740/.
16. L. C. Bailey et al., "Association of Antibiotics in Infancy with Early Childhood Obesity," *JAMA Pediatrics*

168, no. 11 (2014): 1063–69.

17. K. H. Mikkelsen et al., "Use of Antibiotics and Risk of Type 2 Diabetes: A Population-Based Case-Control Study," *Journal of Clinical Endocrinology and Metabolism* 100, no. 10 (2015): 3633–40.
18. A. Hviid et al., "Antibiotic Use and Inflammatory Bowel Diseases in Childhood," *Gut* 60 (2011): 49–54.
19. L. Virta et al., "Association of Repeated Exposure to Antibiotics with the Development of Pediatric Crohn's Disease: A Nationwide, Register-Based Finnish Case-Control Study," *American Journal of Epidemiology* 175, no. 8 (April 15, 2012): 775–84.
20. J. W. Y. Mak et al., "Childhood Antibiotics as a Risk Factor for Crohn's Disease: The ENIGMA International Cohort Study," *Journal of Gastroenterology and Hepatology Open* 6, no. 6 (June 2022): 369–77.
21. E. T. Rogawski et al., *Bulletin of the World Health Organization* 95 (2017): 49–61.
22. Y. Cao et al., "Long-Term Use of Antibiotics and Risk of Colorectal Adenoma," *Gut* 67, no. 4 (2018): 672–78.

23. R. L. Siegel, K. D. Miller, and A. Jemal, "Cancer Statistics, 2017," *CA: A Cancer Journal for Clinicians* 67 (2017): 7–30.
24. M. Zepeda-Rivera et al., "A Distinct *Fusobacterium nucleatum* Clade Dominates the Colorectal Cancer Niche," *Nature* 628 (2024): 424–32.
25. M. C. King et al., "Breast and Ovarian Cancer Risks Due to Inherited Mutations in BRCA1 and BRCA2," *Science* 302, no. 5645 (2003): 643–46.
26. Research in progress by Dr. X. S. Zhang et al., Rutgers University.
27. Research in progress by Dr. Z. Gao et al., Rutgers University.
28. Aversa et al., "Association of Infant Antibiotic Exposure."
29. J. M. Baker, L. Al-Nakkash, and M. M. Herbst-Kralovetz, "Estrogen-Gut Microbiome Axis: Physiological and Clinical Implications," *Maturitas* 103 (September 2017): 45–53.
30. M. G. Dominguez-Bello et al., "Partial Restoration of the Microbiota of Cesarean-Born Infants Via Vaginal Microbial Transfer," *Nature Medicine* 22, no. 3 (March 2016): 250–53.
31. F. Fouhy et al., "Perinatal Factors Affect the Gut Microbiota Up to

Four Years after Birth," *Nature Communications* 10 (April 2019): 1517–10.

32. N. T. Mueller et al., "'Vaginal Seeding' after a Caesarean Section Provides Benefits to Newborn Children: FOR: Does Exposing Caesarean-Delivered Newborns to the Vaginal Microbiome Affect Their Chronic Disease Risk? The Critical Need for Trials of 'Vaginal Seeding' during Caesarean Section," *BJOG: An International Journal of Obstetrics and Gynaecology* 127, no. 2 (January 2020): 301.
33. R. Sommerstein et al., "Antimicrobial Prophylaxis Administration after Umbilical Cord Clamping in Cesarean Section and the Risk of Surgical Site Infection: A Cohort Study with 55,901 Patients," *Antimicrobial Resistance and Infection Control* 9, no. 201 (2020).
34. J. Stokholm et al., "Delivery Mode and Gut Microbial Changes Correlate with an Increased Risk of Childhood Asthma," *Science Translational Medicine* 12, no. 569 (2020), doi:10.1126/scitranslmed.aax9929.
35. Y. Cao et al., "Evaluation of Birth by Cesarean Delivery and Development

of Early-Onset Colorectal Cancer," *JAMA Network Open* 6, no. 4 (2023), doi:10.1001/jamanetworkopen.2023.10316.
36. J. Suez et al., "Personalized Microbiome-Driven Effects of Non-Nutritive Sweeteners on Human Glucose Tolerance," *Cell* 185, no. 18 (September 1, 2022): 3307–28.e19.
37. E. S. Gruber et al., "To Waste or Not to Waste: Questioning Potential Health Risks of Micro- and Nanoplastics with a Focus on Their Ingestion and Potential Carcinogenicity," *Expo Health* 15 (2023): 33–51.
38. B. Walker and S. Lunder, "Pesticides + Poison Gases = Cheap, Year-Round Strawberries," Environmental Working Group, March 20, 2019, https://www.ewg.org/foodnews/strawberries.php.
39. A. Stacy et al., "Infection Trains the Host for Microbiota-Enhanced Resistance to Pathogens," *Cell* 184, no. 3 (February 4, 2021): 615–27.e17.
40. *The Invisible Extinction,* directed by S. Schenck and S. Lawrence (Microbe Media Productions, 2022), Amazon Prime Video, 2023, 85 min.
41. Suez et al., "Personalized Microbiome-Driven Effects."

42. E. V. Nood et al., "Duodenal Infusion of Donor Feces for Recurrent *Clostridium difficile*," *New England Journal of Medicine* 368 (2013): 407–15.
43. F. Dickerson et al., "Adjunctive Probiotic Microorganisms to Prevent Rehospitalization in Patients with Acute Mania: A Randomized Controlled Trial," *Bipolar Disorders* 20, no. 7 (2018): 614–21.
44. P. Feuerstadt, N. Theriault, and G. Tillotson, "The Burden of CDI in the U.S.: A Multifactorial Challenge," *BMC Infectious Diseases* 23 (2023).
45. E. H. Yoo, H. L. Hong, and E. J. Kim, "Epidemiology and Mortality Analysis Related to Carbapenem-Resistant Enterobacterales in Patients after Admission to Intensive Care Units: An Observational Study," *Infection and Drug Resistance* 16 (January 7, 2023): 189–200.
46. Centers for Disease Control and Prevention, *Antibiotic Resistance Threats in the United States, 2019* (Atlanta, GA: U.S. Department of Health and Human Services, Centers for Disease Control, 2019).
47. United Nations Environment Programme, *Bracing for Superbugs:*

Strengthening Environmental Action in the One Health Response to Antimicrobial Resistance, February 7, 2023.

48. M. Drexler, "Seeking the Path of Least Resistance," *Harvard Public Health,* Spring 2019, https://www.hsph.harvard.edu/magazine/magazine_article/seeking-the-path-of-least-resistance/.
49. Information on the Presidential Advisory Council on Combating Antibiotic-Resistant Bacteria is available at https://www.hhs.gov/ash/advisory-committees/paccarb/index.html.

Chapter 4: My Uncle Sam Loves Eggs

1. G. A. Soliman, "Dietary Cholesterol and the Lack of Evidence in Cardiovascular Disease," *Nutrients* 10, no. 6 (June 2018): 780.
2. Guidance was to restrict dietary cholesterol to 300 mg/day.
3. M. Dehghan et al., "Association of Egg Intake with Blood Lipids, Cardiovascular Disease, and Mortality in 177,000 People in 50 Countries," *American Journal of Clinical Nutrition* 111, no. 4 (2020): 795–803.
4. J. Crane et al., "Achievements in

Public Health, 1900–1999," *Morbidity and Mortality Weekly Report* 48, no. 30 (1999).

5. A. Keys and J. T. Anderson, "The Relationship of the Diet to the Development of Atherosclerosis in Man," in *Symposium on Atherosclerosis,* ed. National Research Council, Division of Medical Sciences (Washington, D.C.: National Academy of Sciences — National Research Council, 1954), 181–96.
6. N. Teicholz, "A Short History of Saturated Fat: The Making and Unmaking of a Scientific Consensus," *Current Opinion in Endocrinology, Diabetes and Obesity* 30, no. 1 (February 1, 2023): 65–71.
7. A. Keys, "Atherosclerosis: A Problem in Newer Public Health," *Journal of the Mount Sinai Hospital* 20, no. 2 (July 1953): 118–39, Arthur H. Aufses, Jr., MD Archives, Icahn School of Medicine at Mount Sinai/ Mount Sinai Health System, New York, AA117.S005.SS004.I018, https://archives.mssm.edu/bitstream-7357.
8. N. Healey, "Is There More to a Healthy-Heart Diet than Cholesterol: A High-Fat Diet Is Thought to

Increase the Risk of a Heart Attack. But Some Say the Long-Held Dogma of 'Bad' Cholesterol Might be Flawed," *Scientific American,* November 3, 2021.

9. *Time,* January 13, 1961.
10. C. E. Kearns, L. A. Schmidt, and S. A. Glantz, "Sugar Industry and Coronary Heart Disease Research: A Historical Analysis of Internal Industry Documents," *JAMA Internal Medicine* 176, no. 11 (2016): 1680–85.
11. C. Domonoske, "50 Years Ago, Sugar Industry Quietly Paid Scientists to Point Blame at Fat," NPR, September 13, 2016, www.npr.org/sections/thetwo-way/2016/09/13/493739074/50-years-ago-sugar-industry-quietly-paid-scientists-to-point-blame-at-fat.
12. K. Sarri and A. Kafatos, "The Seven Countries Study in Crete: Olive Oil, Mediterranean Diet or Fasting?" *Public Health Nutrition* 8, no. 6 (September 2005): 666.
13. J. Yerushalmy and H. E. Hilleboe, "Fat in the Diet and Mortality from Heart Disease; a Methodologic Note," *New York State Journal of Medicine* 15, no. 57 (1957): 2343.
14. J. Yudkin, "Dietary Carbohydrate

and Serum-Cholesterol," *Lancet* 303, no. 7864 (1974).
15. Teicholz, "A Short History of Saturated Fat."
16. J. Bowden, "The Biggest Myth & Scientific Deception in Medical History!" *UK Health Radio,* produced by M. Demasi, radio, https://ukhealthradio.com/blog/2013/11/the-biggest-myth-scientific-deception-in-medical-history/.
17. Personal communication with Dr. O. Devinsky.
18. Kearns, Schmidt, and Glantz, "Sugar Industry and Coronary Heart Disease Research."
19. R. B. McGandy, D. M. Hegsted, and F. J. Stare, "Dietary Fats, Carbohydrates and Atherosclerotic Vascular Disease," *New England Journal of Medicine* 255, no. 5 (1967): 245–47.
20. H. Blackburn, "Contrasting Professional Views on Atherosclerosis and Coronary Disease," *New England Journal of Medicine* 292, no. 2 (1975): 105–7.
21. G. Taubes, "What If It's All Been a Big Fat Lie?" *New York Times Magazine,* July 7, 2002.
22. I. D. Frantz Jr. et al., "Test of

Effect of Lipid Lowering by Diet on Cardiovascular Risk. The Minnesota Coronary Survey," *Arteriosclerosis* 9, no. 1 (January–February 1989): 129–35.
23. Personal communication with G. Taubes.
24. Associated Press, "Heart Association to Endorse Some Foods," *New York Times,* June 28, 1988.
25. W. Kannel and T. Gordon, "Section 24: The Framingham Diet Study: Diet and the Regulation of Serum Cholesterol," unpublished data, accessed January 22, 2024, https://www.scribd.com/document/583903774/Kannel-W-Gordon-T-Framingham-dietary-data-Section-24-unpublished.
26. Teicholz, "A Short History of Saturated Fat."
27. Personal communication with Dr. O. Devinsky.
28. B. V. Howard et al., "Low-Fat Dietary Pattern and Risk of Cardiovascular Disease: The Women's Health Initiative Randomized Controlled Dietary Modification Trial," *Journal of the American Medical Association* 295, no. 6 (February 8, 2006): 655–66.
29. C. Purdy and H. B. Evich, "The

Money Behind the Fight over Healthy Eating," *Politico,* October 7, 2015, https://www.politico.com/story/2015/10/the-money-behind-the-fight-over-healthy-eating-214517.
30. I. Oransky, "Obituary: Ancel Keys," *Lancet* 362, no. 9452 (December 18, 2004): 2174.
31. J. E. Brody, "Dr. Ancel Keys, 100, Promoter of the Mediterranean Diet, Died," *New York Times,* November 23, 2004.
32. I. Leslie, "The Sugar Conspiracy," *Guardian,* April 7, 2016.
33. K. M. Flegal et al., "Association of All-Cause Mortality with Overweight and Obesity Using Standard Body Mass Index Categories: A Systematic Review and Meta-Analysis," *Journal of the American Medical Association* 309, no. 1 (2013): 71–82.
34. A. Aubrey, "Research: A Little Extra Fat May Help You Live Longer," NPR, January 2, 2013, https://www.npr.org/sections/health-shots/2013/01/02/168437030/research-a-little-extra-fat-may-help-you-live-longer.
35. K. Flegal, "The Obesity Wars and the Education of a Researcher: A Personal Account," *Progress in Cardiovascular*

Diseases 67, (2021): 75–76.

36. LIPID Study Group (Long-Term Intervention with Pravastatin in Ischaemic Disease), "Long-Term Effectiveness and Safety of Pravastatin in 9014 Patients with Coronary Heart Disease and Average Cholesterol Concentrations: The LIPID Trial Follow-Up," *Lancet* 359, no. 9315 (April 20, 2002): 1379–87.
37. "Dietary Fats," American Heart Association, accessed January 2, 2024, www.heart.org/en/healthy-living/healthy-eating/eat-smart/fats/dietary-fats.

Chapter 5: True Believers

1. J. F. Svensson et al., "Nonoperative Treatment with Antibiotics versus Surgery for Acute Nonperforated Appendicitis in Children: A Pilot Randomized Controlled Trial," *Annals of Surgery* 261, no. 1 (2015): 67–71.
2. P. Salminen et al., "Antibiotic Therapy vs Appendectomy for Treatment of Uncomplicated Acute Appendicitis: The APPAC Randomized Clinical Trial," *Journal of the American Medical Association* 313, no. 23 (2015): 2340–48.

3. H. C. Park et al., "Randomized Clinical Trial of Antibiotic Therapy for Uncomplicated Appendicitis," *British Journal of Surgery* 104, no. 13 (2017): 1785–90.
4. P. Salminen et al., "Five-Year Follow-Up of Antibiotic Therapy for Uncomplicated Acute Appendicitis in the APPAC Randomized Clinical Trial," *Journal of the American Medical Association* 320, no. 12 (2018): 1259–65.
5. Svensson et al., "Nonoperative Treatment with Antibiotics versus Surgery for Acute Nonperforated Appendicitis in Children."
6. P. C. Minneci et al., "Association of Nonoperative Management Using Antibiotic Therapy vs Laparoscopic Appendectomy with Treatment Success and Disability Days in Children with Uncomplicated Appendicitis," *Journal of the American Medical Association* 324, no. 6 (August 11, 2020): 581–93.
7. L. Festinger and J. M. Carlsmith, "Cognitive Consequences of Forced Compliance," *Journal of Abnormal and Social Psychology* 58, no. 2 (1959): 203–10.
8. E. Aronson and J. Mills, "The Effect

of Severity of Initiation on Liking for a Group," *Journal of Abnormal and Social Psychology* 59, no. 2 (1959): 177–81.
9. L. Festinger, H. Riecken, and S. Schachter, *When Prophecy Fails: A Social and Psychological Study of a Modern Group that Predicted the Destruction of the World* (Minneapolis: University of Minnesota Press, 1954; repr., New York: Harper Torchbooks, 1964).
10. Ibid.
11. Ibid.

Chapter 6: Bad Blood

1. Institute of Medicine, Committee to Study HIV Transmission through Blood and Blood Products, *HIV and the Blood Supply: An Analysis of Crisis Decisionmaking,* ed. L. B. Leveton, H. C. Cox Jr., and M. A. Stoto (Washington, D.C.: National Academies Press, 1995).
2. R. C. Adams and J. S. Lundy, "Anesthesia in Cases of Poor Surgical Risk: Some Suggestions for Decreasing the Risk," *Anesthesiology* 3 (1942): 603–7.
3. C. Madjdpour and D. R. Spahn, "Allogeneic Red Blood Cell

Transfusions: Efficacy, Risks, Alternatives and Indications," *British Journal of Anaesthesia* 95, no. 1 (July 2005): 33–42.

4. R. P. Dellinger et al. and the Surviving Sepsis Campaign Guidelines Committee including the Pediatric Subgroup, "Surviving Sepsis Campaign: International Guidelines for Management of Severe Sepsis and Septic Shock, 2012," *Intensive Care Medicine* 39, no. 2 (February 2013): 165–228.
5. A. Shander et al. and the International Consensus Conference on Transfusion Outcomes Group, "Appropriateness of Allogeneic Red Blood Cell Transfusion: The International Consensus Conference on Transfusion Outcomes," *Transfusion Medicine Reviews* 25, no. 3 (July 2011): 232–46.e53.
6. Institute of Medicine, *HIV and the Blood Supply.*
7. *Federal Response to AIDS: Hearings Before a Subcommittee of the Committee on Government Operations, U.S. House of Representatives, Ninety-Eighth Congress, August 1–2, 1983* (Washington, D.C.: U.S. Government Printing Office, 1983), 629.

8. Ibid., 294.
9. Ibid., 165.
10. Ibid., 235.
11. Ibid., 242.
12. A. S. Fauci, *AIDS: Acquired Immunodeficiency Syndrome* (Bethesda, MD: National Institutes of Health Clinical Center, 1984), film, 60. min, http://resource.nlm.nih.gov/101674642.
13. C. Wallis, "Battling AIDS," *Time,* April 29, 1985.
14. Institute of Medicine, *HIV and the Blood Supply.*
15. R. Richter, "Blood Quest: The Battle to Protect Transfusions from HIV," in "Blood at Work: What Do We Know about It?" special issue, *Stanford Medicine,* Spring 2013.
16. Institute of Medicine, *HIV And The Blood Supply.*
17. S. Stolberg, "Column One: Cruel Link: Hemophilia and AIDS: Transfusions that Once Were Seen as a Salvation Brought a Deadly Epidemic in the 1980s. After a Decade of Anguish and Frustration, Survivors Are Fighting Back," *Los Angeles Times,* August 31, 1994.
18. California Senate Bill No. 1419, Chapter 888, https://leginfo.legislature

.ca.gov/faces/billTextClient.xhtml?bill_id=202120220SB1419.
19. California Medical Association, "Governor signs CMA-sponsored bill giving physicians time to interpret test results for patients," news release, October 3, 2022, https://www.cmadocs.org/newsroom/news/view/ArticleID/49898/t/Governor-signs-CMA-sponsored-bill-160-giving-physicians-time-to-interpret-test-results-for-patients.
20. Richter, "Blood Quest."
21. L. J. Altman, "The Doctor's World: C.D.C. Is Embarrassed by Its Tardy Response to AIDS-Like Illness," *New York Times,* July 28, 1992.
22. Ibid.
23. U. L. McFarling, "When a Cardiologist Flagged the Lack of Diversity at Premier Medical Journals, the Silence Was Telling," Stat, April 12, 2021, https://www.statnews.com/2021/04/12/lack-of-diversity-at-premier-medical-journals-jama-nejm/.
24. B. Blanchard, "China's Blood Still Unsafe, Needs Help: Report," Reuters, September 6, 2007, https://www.reuters.com/article/idUSPEK333640/.
25. "Contaminated Needles Spread

Hepatitis in China," Infection Control Today, August 10, 2001, https://www.infectioncontroltoday.com/view/contaminated-needles-spread-hepatitis-china.
26. R. D. Eckert, "The AIDS Blood-Transfusion Cases: A Legal and Economic Analysis of Liability," *San Diego Law Review* 29, no. 203 (1992): 206.
27. Ibid.
28. Ibid.
29. J. Thomas et al., "Anemia and Blood Transfusion Practices in the Critically Ill: A Prospective Cohort Review," *Heart and Lung* 39, no. 3 (May–June 2010): 217–25.
30. A. Kaplan et al., "Informed Consent for Blood Transfusion," Association for the Advancement of Blood and Biotherapies, February 23, 2023, https://www.aabb.org/docs/default-source/default-document-library/resources/informed-consent-for-blood-transfusion.pdf?sfvrsn=b2ee9851_2.
31. Eckert, "The AIDS Blood-Transfusion Cases," 219–20.
32. M. K. F. Salamat et al., "Preclinical Transmission of Prions by Blood Transfusion Is Influenced by

Donor Genotype and Route of Infection," *PLOS Pathogens* 17, no. 2 (February 18, 2021), doi:10.1371/journal.ppat.1009276.

33. E. P. Winer, presidential address, American Society of Clinical Oncology Annual Meeting, Chicago, IL, and online, June 2–6, 2023.

Chapter 7: A Warm Welcome

1. L. V. Simon, M. F. Hashmi, and B. N. Bragg, APGAR Score [updated May 22, 2023], in *StatPearls* (Treasure Island, FL: StatPearls Publishing, January 2024), https://www.ncbi.nlm.nih.gov/books/NBK470569/.
2. F. R. Greer, "Feeding the Premature Infant in the 20th Century," in "Symposium: Accomplishments in Child Nutrition during the 20th Century," ed. B. L. Nichols and F. R. Greer, supp., *Journal of Nutrition* 131, no. 2 (February 2001): 426S–30S.
3. A. Patz, L. E. Hoeck, and E. De La Cruz, "Studies on the Effect of High Oxygen Administration in Retrolental Fibroplasia: I. Nursery Observations," *American Journal of Ophthalmology* 35 (1952): 1248–53.
4. E. Naumburg et al., "Supplementary

Oxygen and Risk of Childhood Lymphatic Leukaemia," *Acta Paediatrica* 91, no. 12 (2002): 1328–33.
5. S. Rovner, "Surgery Without Anesthesia: Can Preemies Feel Pain?" *Washington Post,* August 13, 1986.
6. J. H. Hess and E. C. Lundeen, *The Premature Infant: Its Medical and Nursing Care* (Philadelphia: J. B. Lippincott, 1941), 99–153.
7. J. Gleiss, "ZumFrühgeborenenproblem der Gegenwart IX. Mitteilung. Über fütterungs–und unweltbedignte Atemstörungen bei Frühgeborenen," *Zeitschrift für Kinderheilkunde* 76 (1955): 261–68.
8. J. D. L. Hansen and C. A. Smith, "Effects of Withholding Fluid in the Immediate Postnatal Period," *Pediatrics* 12 (1953): 99–113.
9. M. Singata, J. Tranmer, and G. M. Gyte, "Restricting Oral Fluid and Food Intake During Labour," *Cochrane Database of Systematic Reviews* 8 (August 22, 2013), doi:10.1002/14651858.CD003930.pub3.
10. A. Chiruvolu et al., "Effect of Delayed Cord Clamping on Very Preterm Infants," *American Journal of Obstetrics and Gynecology* 213, no. 5 (2015): 676.

11. A. Chiruvolu et al., "Effect of Delayed Cord Clamping on Very Preterm Twins," *Early Human Development* 124 (2018): 22–25.
12. A. Chiruvolu et al., "The Effect of Delayed Cord Clamping on Moderate and Early Late-Preterm Infants," *American Journal of Perinatology* 35, no. 3 (2018): 286–91.
13. A. Chiruvolu et al., "Effects of Umbilical Cord Milking on Term Infants Delivered by Cesarean Section," *American Journal of Perinatology* 38, no. 10 (2021): 1042–2047.
14. Ibid.
15. Chiruvolu et al., "Effect of Delayed Cord Clamping on Very Preterm Twins."
16. R. M. Soliman et al., "A Randomized Controlled Trial of a 30- Versus a 120-Second Delay in Cord Clamping after Term Birth," *American Journal of Perinatology* (March 11, 2022).
17. A. L. Seidler et al. and iCOMP Collaborators, "Deferred Cord Clamping, Cord Milking, and Immediate Cord Clamping at Preterm Birth: A Systematic Review and Individual Participant Data

Meta-Analysis," *Lancet* 402, no. 10418 (December 9, 2023): 2209–22.

18. University of Sydney, "Delaying Cord Clamping Could Halve Risk of Death in Premature Babies," news release, November 15, 2023.
19. J. S. Mercer et al., "The Effects of Delayed Cord Clamping on 12-Month Brain Myelin Content and Neurodevelopment: A Randomized Controlled Trial," *American Journal of Perinatology* 39, no. 1 (January 2022): 37–44.
20. "What Is Kangaroo Care and How Can It Help Your Baby?" Cleveland Clinic, accessed January 13, 2024, https://my.clevelandclinic.org/health/treatments/12578-kangaroo-care.
21. A. Whitelaw and K. Sleath, "Myth of the Marsupial Mother: Home Care of Very Low Birth Weight Babies in Bogota, Colombia," *Lancet* 1, no. 8439 (May 25, 1985): 1206–8.
22. N. J. Bergman and L. A. Jürisoo, "The 'Kangaroo-Method' for Treating Low Birth Weight Babies in a Developing Country," *Tropical Doctor* 24, no. 2 (April 1994): 57–60.
23. A. Chiruvolu et al., "Effects of Skin-to-Skin Care on Late Preterm and

Term Infants At-Risk for Neonatal Hypoglycemia," *Pediatric Quality and Safety* 2, no. 4 (June 20, 2017), doi:10.1097/pq9.0000000000000030.

24. A. E. de Alencar et al., "Effect of Kangaroo Mother Care on Postpartum Depression," *Journal of Tropical Pediatrics* 55, no. 1 (February 2009): 36–38.
25. E. R. Moore et al., "Early Skin-to-Skin Contact for Mothers and Their Healthy Newborn Infants," *Cochrane Database of Systematic Reviews* 11 (2016), doi:10.1002/14651858.CD003519.pub4.
26. Chiruvolu et al., "Effects of Skin-to-Skin Care on Late Preterm and Term Infants."
27. World Health Organization, "Kangaroo Mother Care: A Transformative Innovation in Health Care" (global position paper; Geneva: World Health Organization, 2023), license: CC BY-NC-SA 3.0 IGO.
28. D. D. Flannery et al., "Temporal Trends and Center Variation in Early Antibiotic Use Among Premature Infants," *JAMA Network Open* 1, no. 1 (May 18, 2018), doi:10.1001/jamanetworkopen.2018.0164.

29. N. T. Mueller et al., " 'Vaginal Seeding' after a Caesarean Section Provides Benefits to Newborn Children: FOR: Does Exposing Caesarean-Delivered Newborns to the Vaginal Microbiome Affect Their Chronic Disease Risk? The Critical Need for Trials of 'Vaginal Seeding' during Caesarean Section," *BJOG: An International Journal of Obstetrics and Gynaecology* 127, no. 2 (January 2020): 301.
30. E. L. Rudey, M. D. C. Leal, and G. Rego, "Cesarean Section Rates in Brazil: Trend Analysis Using the Robson Classification System," *Medicine* (Baltimore) 99, no. 17 (April 2020), doi:10.1097/MD.0000000000019880.
31. J. G. Albertini et al., "Evaluation of a Peer-to-Peer Data Transparency Intervention for Mohs Micrographic Surgery Overuse," *JAMA Dermatology* 155, no. 8 (August 1, 2019): 906–13.
32. K. K. Hoppe and B. Bosse, "Complicated Deliveries," in *Avery's Diseases of the Newborn,* 11th ed., ed. C. A. Gleason and T. Sawyer (Philadelphia: Elsevier, 2024), 135–46.e2.

33. National Institute of Child Health and Human Development, Maternal-Fetal Medicine Units Network, vaginal birth after cesarean online calculator, version 2.2, updated November 2023, https://mfmunetwork.bsc.gwu.edu/web/mfmunetwork/vaginal-birth-after-cesarean-calculator.
34. Ibid.
35. W. A. Grobman et al., "Labor Induction Versus Expectant Management in Low-Risk Nulliparous Women," *New England Journal of Medicine* 379 (2018): 513–23.
36. E. Nethery et al., "Effects of the ARRIVE (A Randomized Trial of Induction Versus Expectant Management) Trial on Elective Induction and Obstetric Outcomes in Term Nulliparous Patients," *Obstetrics and Gynecology* 142, no. 2 (August 11, 2023): 242–50.
37. P. J. Meis et al. and the National Institute of Child Health and Human Development Maternal-Fetal Medicine Units Network, "Prevention of Recurrent Preterm Delivery by 17 Alpha-Hydroxyprogesterone Caproate," *New England Journal of Medicine* 348, no. 24 (June 12, 2003): 2379–85.

Erratum in *New England Journal of Medicine* 349, no. 13 (September 25, 2003): 1299.

38. U.S. Food and Drug Administration, "FDA Commissioner and Chief Scientist Announce Decision to Withdraw Approval of Makena," press release, April 6, 2023.
39. Centers for Disease Control and Prevention, "Achievements in Public Health, 1900–1999: Healthier Mothers and Babies," *Morbidity and Mortality Weekly Report* 48, no. 38 (October 1999): 849–58.

Chapter 8: Challenging Certainty

1. American Cancer Society, "Key Statistics for Ovarian Cancer," last revised October 3, 2023, https://www.cancer.org/cancer/types/ovarian-cancer/about/key-statistics.html.
2. S. Kyo et al., "The Fallopian Tube as Origin of Ovarian Cancer: Change of Diagnostic and Preventive Strategies," *Cancer Medicine* 9, no. 2 (January 2020): 421–31, doi:10.1002/cam4.2725.
3. L. Dubeau, "The Cell of Origin of Ovarian Epithelial Tumors and the Ovarian Surface Epithelium Dogma:

Does the Emperor Have No Clothes?" *Gynecologic Oncology* 72, no. 3 (1999): 437–42.
4. J. M. Piek et al., "Dysplastic Changes in Prophylactically Removed Fallopian Tubes of Women Predisposed to Developing Ovarian Cancer," *Journal of Pathology* 195, no. 4 (2001): 451–56.
5. F. Medeiros et al., "The Tubal Fimbria Is a Preferred Site for Early Adenocarcinoma in Women with Familial Ovarian Cancer Syndrome," *American Journal of Surgical Pathology* 30, no. 2 (February 2006): 230–36.
6. S. Labidi-Galy et al., "High Grade Serous Ovarian Carcinomas Originate in the Fallopian Tube," *Nature Communications* 8, no. 1093 (2017).
7. American College of Obstetricians and Gynecologists, Committee on Gynecologic Practice, "Opportunistic Salpingectomy as a Strategy for Epithelial Ovarian Cancer Prevention," ACOG Committee Opinion No. 774, in *Obstetrics and Gynecology* 133, no. 4 (April 2019), doi:10.1097/AOG.00000 0000003164.
8. Ibid.
9. A. C. Restaino et al., "Functional Neuronal Circuits Promote Disease

Progression in Cancer," *Science Advances* 9, no. 19 (May 10, 2023), doi: 10.1126/sciadv.ade4443.
10. H. D. Reavis, H. I. Chen, and R. Drapkin, "Tumor Innervation: Cancer Has Some Nerve," *Trends in Cancer* 6, no. 12 (December 2020): 1059–67.
11. G. Hanley, "Presentation to the American Academy of Cancer Research Special Conference in Cancer Research: Ovarian Cancer," Boston, October 6, 2023.
12. R. M. Kahn et al., "Salpingectomy for the Primary Prevention of Ovarian Cancer," *JAMA Surgery* (September 6, 2023).
13. V. Giannakeas et al., "Salpingectomy and the Risk of Ovarian Cancer in Ontario," *JAMA Network Open* 6, no. 8 (August 1, 2023), doi:10.1001/jamanetworkopen.2023.27198.
14. I. C. Cook and C. N. Landen, "Opportunistic Salpingectomy in Women Undergoing Non-Gynecologic Abdominal Surgery," *Gynecologic Oncology* 158, no. 1 (2020), doi:10.1016/j.ygyno.2020.04.005.
15. R. Sowamber et al., "Ovarian Cancer: From Precursor Lesion Identification to Population-Based Prevention

Programs," *Current Oncology* 30, no. 12 (November 29, 2023): 10179–94.

16. R. Stone, J. V. Sakran, and K. Long Roche, "Salpingectomy in Ovarian Cancer Prevention," *Journal of the American Medical Association* 329, no. 23 (June 20, 2023): 2015–16.
17. N. Nabavi, "Screening for Ovarian Cancer Is Ruled Out after Trial Found It Did Not Reduce Deaths," *BMJ: British Medical Journal* 373 (2021): n1223.
18. C. J. Cabasag et al., "Ovarian Cancer Today and Tomorrow: A Global Assessment by World Region and Human Development Index Using GLOBOCAN 2020," *International Journal of Cancer* 151, no. 9 (November 1, 2022): 1535–41.
19. R. Drapkin, "Progress in Ovarian Cancer: Discovery of Fallopian Tube Involvement," MDedge, June 26, 2023, https://www.mdedge.com/hematology-oncology/article/263338/ovarian-cancer/progress-ovarian-cancer-discovery-fallopian-tube.
20. National Human Genome Research Institute, "Eugenics: Its Origin and Development (1883–Present)," accessed

April 2, 2024, https://www.genome.gov/about-genomics/educational-resources/timelines/eugenics.

21. S. P. Raine, "Federal Sterilization Policy: Unintended Consequences," *American Medical Association Journal of Ethics, Virtual Mentor* 14, no. 2 (February 2012): 152–57, https://journalofethics.ama-assn.org/article/federal-sterilization-policy-unintended-consequences/2012-02.
22. Ñ. C. Ko, "Peru's Government Forcibly Sterilized Indigenous Women from 1996 to 2001, the Women Say. Why?" *Washington Post,* February 19, 2021.
23. "Peru Forced Sterilisations Case Reaches Key Stage," BBC News, March 1, 2021, https://www.bbc.com/news/world-latin-america-56201575.
24. D. Anderson et al., "Feasibility of Opportunistic Salpingectomy at the Time of a vNOTES Hysterectomy: A Retrospective Cohort," *International Journal of Gynecology and Obstetrics* 163, no. 3 (December 2023): 1026–27.

Chapter 9: Silicone Valley

1. R. R. Cook and L. L. Perkins, "The Prevalence of Breast Implants Among

Women in the United States," *Current Topics in Microbiology and Immunology* 210 (1996): 419–25.

2. *Face to Face with Connie Chung,* episode aired December 10, 1990, on CBS.
3. "CBS Cancels Ad Decrying Connie Chung Report on Breast Implants," United Press International, November 9, 1991, https://www.upi.com/Archives/1991/11/09/CBS-cancels-ad-decrying-Connie-Chung-report-on-breast-implants/8141689662800/.
4. D. E. Bernstein, "Review: The Breast Implant Fiasco," *California Law Review* 87, no. 2 (1999): 457–510.
5. K. E. Schleiter, "Silicone Breast Implant Litigation," *American Medical Association Journal of Ethics, Virtual Mentor* 12, no. 5 (2010): 389–94, https://journalofethics.ama-assn.org/article/silicone-breast-implant-litigation/2010-05.
6. "Breast Implants Riskier than FDA Admits, Lawmaker Says," *Tampa Bay Times,* April 28, 2005.
7. P. J. Hilts, "FDA Seeks Halt in Breast Implants Made of Silicone," *New York Times,* January 7, 1992.
8. S. A. Van Nunen, P. A. Gatenby, and A. Basten, "Post-Mammoplasty

Connective Tissue Disease," *Arthritis and Rheumatism* 25 (1982): 694–97.
9. D. A. Kessler, "The Basis of the FDA's Decision on Breast Implants," *New England Journal of Medicine* 326, no. 25 (June 18, 1992): 1713–15.
10. Ibid.
11. S. Roan, "Time Not on Their Side, Say Women with Implants: Health: Angry and Scared, They Say They Cannot Afford to Wait Until Late 1994 for the Results of Government Studies," *Los Angeles Times,* May 18, 1993.
12. U.S. Government Accountability Office Human Resources Division letter to Congressman Donald M. Payne, December 7, 1992.
13. Z. S. F. Lam and D. Hurry, "Dow Corning and the Silicone Implant Controversy" (working paper, Southern Methodist University Cox School of Business, January 1, 1992), https://scholar.smu.edu/cgi/viewcontent.cgi?article=1155&context=business_workingpapers.
14. M. Angell, "Breast Implants: Protection or Paternalism?" *New England Journal of Medicine* 326 (June 18, 1992): 1695–96.

15. D. A. Kessler, R. B., Merkatz, and R. Schapiro, "A Call for Higher Standards for Breast Implants," *Journal of the American Medical Association* 270, no. 21 (December 1, 1993): 2607–8, PMID: 8230647.
16. U.S. Food and Drug Administration, "Timeline of Selected FDA Activities and Significant Events Addressing Substance Use and Overdose Prevention," accessed February 14, 2025, www.fda.gov/drugs/information-drug-class/timeline-selected-fda-activities-and-significant-events-addressing-substance-use-and-overdose.
17. Ibid.
18. Sam Hornblower, "How the FDA Supercharged the Opioid Epidemic," The Conversation, in press, 2024.
19. J. Porter and H. Jick, "Addiction Rare in Patients Treated with Narcotics," *New England Journal of Medicine* 302, no. 2 (January 10, 1980): 123.
20. C. Brummett et al., "New Persistent Opioid Use After Minor and Major Surgical Procedures in U.S. Adults," *JAMA Surgery* 152, no. 6 (2017).
21. M. Allen and A. Richards, "The New Addiction: The Painful Truth

about Nevada: Many Nevadans Crave Painkillers, and Some Doctors Oblige," *Las Vegas Sun,* July 6, 2008.
22. Schleiter, "Silicone Breast Implant Litigation."
23. Wired Staff, "Implant Settlement," *Wired,* July 8, 1998.
24. S. E. Gabriel et al., "Risk of Connective-Tissue Diseases and Other Disorders after Breast Implantation," *New England Journal of Medicine* 330 (1994): 1697–702.
25. L. A. Brinton and S. L. Brown, "Breast Implants and Cancer," *Journal of the National Cancer Institute* 89, no. 18 (September 17, 1997): 1341–49.
26. "25 Most Influential Americans," *Time,* June 24, 2001.
27. D. A. Kessler, in response to M. Angell, "Breast Implants — Protection or Paternalism?" *New England Journal of Medicine* 326, no. 25 (June 18, 1992):1695–96, comments accessed December 28, 2023, doi:10.1056/NEJM199206183262510, PMID:1588985.
28. P. A. McGuire et al., "Separating Myth from Reality in Breast Implants: An Overview of 30 Years of Experience," *Plastic and Reconstructive Surgery* 152,

no. 5 (November 2023): 801e–7e, doi:10.1097/PRS.0000000000010488.
29. Ibid.
30. "Silicone Breast Implants and Cancer," in Institute of Medicine, Committee on the Safety of Silicone Breast Implants, *Safety of Silicone Breast Implants,* ed. S. Bondurant, V. Ernster, and R. Herdman (Washington, D.C.: National Academies Press, 1999).
31. G. Kolata, "In Implant Case, Science and the Law Have Different Agendas," *New York Times,* July 11, 1998.
32. E. Lichtblau and S. Shan, "Vast F.D.A. Effort Tracked E-Mails of Its Scientists," *New York Times,* July 14, 2012.
33. K. Perry, "Disgraced Lawyer Decides to Retire, Not Fight," *Cincinnati Enquirer,* April 19, 2013, https://www.usatoday.com/story/news/nation/2013/04/19/disbarred-lawyer-stanley-chesley/2098107/.
34. A. Head, "You'll Not See Nothing Like the Mighty O'Quinn," *Texas Super Lawyers,* September 22, 2004, https://www.superlawyers.com/articles/texas/youll-not-see-nothing-like-the-mighty-oquinn/.
35. D. C. Weiss, "Lawyer O'Quinn

Ordered to Pay $41.4 M," *ABA Journal,* September 12, 2007, https://www.abajournal.com/news/article/lawyer_oquinn_ordered_to_pay_414_m.
36. Associated Press, "John O'Quinn Dies at 68; Texas Personal-Injury Lawyer," *Los Angeles Times,* October 30, 2009, https://www.latimes.com/local/obituaries/la-me-john-oquinn30-2009oct30-story.html.
37. C. McGreal, "Biden Urged Not to Give Top FDA Job to Official Over Her Role in Opioid Crisis," *Guardian,* January 28, 2021.

Chapter 10: A Comedy of Errors

1. B. Rigas, C. Feretis, and E. D. Papavassiliou, "John Lykoudis: An Unappreciated Discoverer of the Cause and Treatment of Peptic Ulcer Disease," *Lancet* 354, no. 9190 (November 6, 1999): 1634–35.
2. G. Friedland, "Discovery of the Function of the Heart and Circulation of Blood," *Cardiovascular Journal of Africa* 20, no. 3 (May–June 2009): 160, PMID:19575077, PMCID:PMC3721262.
3. B. Hernández, "This English Doctor Upended Everything We Knew

about the Human Heart," *National Geographic,* February 13, 2018, https://www.nationalgeographic.co.uk/science/2018/02/this-english-doctor-upended-everything-we-knew-about-the-human-heart.
4. D. Ribatti, "William Harvey and the Discovery of the Circulation of the Blood," *Journal of Angiogenes Research* 1 (September 2009): 3, doi:10.1186/2040-2384-1-3, PMID:19946411, PMCID:PMC2776239.
5. L. Payne, " 'With Much Nausea, Loathing and Foetor,' William Harvey, Dissection, and Dispassion in Early Modern Medicine," *Vesalius* 8, no. 2 (December 2002): 45–52.
6. G. Friedland and M. Friedman, *Medicine's 10 Greatest Discoveries* (New Haven: Yale University Pres, 1998).
7. M. White, "James Lind: The Man Who Helped to Cure Scurvy with Lemons," BBC News, October 4, 2016, https://www.bbc.com/news/uk-england-37320399.
8. C. Price, "The Age of Scurvy," *Distillations Magazine,* August 14, 2017, https://www.sciencehistory.org/stories/magazine/the-age-of-scurvy/.
9. C. P. McCord, "Scurvy As an

Occupational Disease: VIII. Scurvy and the Slave Trade," *Journal of Occupational Medicine* 14, no. 1 (January 1972): 45–49.
10. I. Milne, "Who Was James Lind, and What Exactly Did He Achieve?" *JLL Bulletin: Commentaries on the History of Treatment Evaluation* (2012), https://www.jameslindlibrary.org/articles/who-was-james-lind-and-what-exactly-did-he-achieve/
11. Ibid.
12. Ibid.
13. A. M. Behbehani, "The Smallpox Story: Life and Death of an Old Disease," *Microbiological Reviews* 47, no. 4 (December 1983): 455–509.
14. K. B. Patterson and T. Runge, "Smallpox and the Native American," *American Journal of the Medical Sciences* 323, no. 4 (April 2002): 216–22.
15. K. A. Smith, "Edward Jenner and the Small Pox Vaccine," *Frontiers in Immunology* 14, no. 2 (June 2011): 21.
16. N. J. Willis, "Edward Jenner and the Eradication of Smallpox," *Scottish Medical Journal* 42, no. 4 (August 1997): 118–21.
17. J. Cassels, "Edward Jenner and the

Cuckoo," Arran Birding, accessed January 8, 2024, www.arranbirding.co.uk/edward-jenner-and-the-cuckoo.html.

18. E. Jenner, *An Inquiry into the Causes and Effects of the Variolae Vaccinae: A Disease Discovered in Some of the Western Counties of England, Particularly Gloucestershire, and Known by the Name of the Cow Pox* (Springfield, MA: Samuel Cooley, 1801).
19. B. S. Leavell, "Thomas Jefferson and Smallpox Vaccination," *Transactions of the American Clinical and Climatological Association* 88 (1977): 119–127.
20. "History of the Smallpox Vaccination," World Health Organization, accessed February 10, 2024, https://www.who.int/news-room/spotlight/history-of-vaccination/history-of-smallpox-vaccination.
21. H. Ellis, "Ignaz Semmelweis: Tragic Pioneer in the Prevention of Puerperal Sepsis," *British Journal of Hospital Medicine* 69, no. 6 (June 2008): 358, doi:10.12968/hmed.2008.69.6.29631, PMID:18646425.
22. P. Rangappa, "Ignaz Semmelweis — Hand Washing Pioneer," *Journal of the Association of Physicians of India* 58

(May 2010): 328, PMID:21117357.

23. I. Loudon, "Ignaz Phillip Semmelweis' Studies of Death in Childbirth," *Journal of the Royal Society of Medicine* 106, no. 11 (November 2013): 461–63.
24. National Research Council, Committee to Update Science, Medicine, and Animals, "A Theory of Germs" in *Science, Medicine, and Animals* (Washington, D.C.: National Academies Press, 2004), 7–8.
25. A. D. Ataman, E. E. Vatanoğlu-Lutz, and G. Yildirim, "Medicine in Stamps: Ignaz Semmelweis and Puerperal Fever," *Journal of the Turkish-German Gynecological Association* 14, no. 1 (March 1, 2013): 35–9.
26. H. Ellis, "Ignaz Semmelweis," 358.
27. G. Zuckerman, "After Shunning Scientist, University of Pennsylvania Celebrates Her Nobel Prize: School That Once Demoted Katalin Karikó and Cut Her Pay Has Made Millions of Dollars from Patenting Her Work," *Wall Street Journal,* October 4, 2023.
28. A. Shrikant, "Nobel Prize Winner Katalin Karikó Was 'Demoted 4 Times' at Her Old Job. How She Persisted: 'You Have to Focus on What's Next,' " CNBC,

October 6, 2023, https://www.cnbc.com/2023/10/06/nobel-prize-winner-katalin-karik-on-being-demoted-perseverance-.html.

29. B. Binday, "'Not of Faculty Quality': How Penn Mistreated Nobel Prize–Winning Researcher Katalin Karikó," *Daily Pennsylvanian,* October 26, 2023.
30. Zuckerman, "After Shunning Scientist, University of Pennsylvania Celebrates Her Nobel Prize."
31. Ibid.
32. "Katalin Karikó and Drew Weissman, Penn's Historic mRNA Vaccine Research Team, Win 2023 Nobel Prize in Medicine," *Penn Today,* October 2, 2023, https://penntoday.upenn.edu/news/katalin-kariko-and-drew-weissman-penns-historic-mrna-vaccine-research-team-win-2023-nobel.

Chapter 11: A Culture of Obedience

1. Murthy v. Missouri, No. 23–411, 2023 U.S. App. (5th Cir. 2023), https://www.supremecourt.gov/DocketPDF/23/23-411/294091/20231222102540387_FINAL%20Murthy%20Amicus%20for%20filing.pdf.
2. J. Swerdin, L. Smaliak, and S.

Niederman, "California Repeals Law Preventing Spread Of Misinformation Regarding Covid-19," The Free Speech Project, Georgetown University, accessed February 7, 2024, http://freespeechproject.georgetown.edu/tracker-entries/ninth-circuit-hears-arguments-on-california-law-punishing-doctors-for-spreading-false-information-about-covid-19.
3. A. Chen and J. Wosen, "Dana-Farber Expands Studies to Be Retracted to 6, Plus 31 to Be Corrected Over Mishandled Data," *Boston Globe,* January 22, 2024.
4. S. David, "Dana-Farberications at Harvard University," *For Better Science* (blog), January 2, 2024, https://forbetterscience.com/2024/01/02/dana-farberications-at-harvard-university/.
5. V. H. Paulus and A. Ravi, "Top Harvard Medical School Neuroscientist Accused of Research Misconduct," *Harvard Crimson,* February 1, 2024.
6. W. L. Wang, "Brigham and Women's Hospital to Pay $10 Million for Research Fraud Allegations," *Harvard Crimson,* April 28, 2017.
7. R. Van Noorden, "More than 10,000 Research Papers Were Retracted in

2023 — A New Record," *Nature,* December 12, 2023, https://www.nature.com/articles/d41586-023-03974-8.

8. R. Sohn, "Exclusive: Committee Recommended Pulling Several Papers by Former Cornell Med School Dean," *Retraction Watch* (blog), March 29, 2023, https://retractionwatch.com/2023/03/29/exclusive-committee-recommended-pulling-several-papers-by-former-cornell-med-school-dean/.
9. David, "Dana-Farberications at Harvard University."
10. J. B. Carlisle, "False Individual Patient Data and Zombie Randomised Controlled Trials Submitted to *Anaesthesia,*" *Anaesthesia* 76, no. 4 (April 2021): 472–79.
11. D. Herrera-Perez et al., "A Comprehensive Review of Randomized Clinical Trials in Three Medical Journals Reveals 396 Medical Reversals," *eLife* 8 (June 11, 2019), doi:10.7554/eLife.45183.
12. "Tamiflu and Relenza: Getting the Full Evidence Picture," Cochrane, accessed February 7, 2024, https://www.cochrane.org/news/tamiflu-and-relenza-getting-full-evidence-picture.

13. T. Jefferson, "The Tamiflu Story: Why We Need Access to All Data from Clinical Trials," *Open Knowledge* (blog), November 19, 2012, https://blog.okfn.org/2012/11/19/the-tamiflu-story-why-we-need-access-to-all-data-from-clinical-trials.
14. Z. Damania and V. Prasad, "CDC Masking Comments, Prior Auths, Paxlovid Data," *The VPZD Show* (podcast), February 15, 2023, https://zdoggmd.com/vpzd-31/.
15. E. M. Bik, A. Casadevall, and F. C. Fang, "The Prevalence of Inappropriate Image Duplication in Biomedical Research Publications," *mBio* 7, no. 3 (June 2016), doi:10.1128/mBio.00809-16.
16. A. Marcus and I. Oransky, "A Rash of Scientific Retraction," *Boston Globe,* April 17, 2012.
17. G. Kolata, "In a First, *New England Journal of Medicine* Joins Never-Trumpers," *New York Times,* October 7, 2020.
18. "Dying in a Leadership Vacuum," editorial, *New England Journal of Medicine* 383 (October 8, 2020): 1479–80, https://www.nejm.org/doi/full/10.1056/NEJMe2029812.

19. "Should *Nature* Endorse Political Candidates: Yes, When the Occasion Demands It," editorial, *Nature,* March 20, 2020, https://www.nature.com/articles/d41586-023-00789-5.
20. M. Makary et al., "Prevalence and Durability of SARS-CoV-2 Antibodies Among Unvaccinated U.S. Adults by History of COVID-19," *JAMA Network* 327, no. 11 (February 3, 2022): 1085–87, https://jamanetwork.com/journals/jama/fullarticle/2788894.
21. "Most Viewed Articles: 2022," *Journal of the American Medical Association,* accessed March 18, 2024, https://jamanetwork.com/pages/2022-most-discussed-articles.
22. "The Cancellation of Leana Wen," editorial, *Wall Street Journal,* August 23, 2022.
23. S. Siles, "STS, New President Apologize for Predecessor's Speech Amid Twitter Backlash," Medscape, January 26, 2023, https://www.medscape.com/viewarticle/987571?form=fpf.
24. Warren Newton, Richard J. Baron, and David G. Nichols, "Joint Statement on Dissemination of Information," American Board of Internal Medicine,

accessed April 28, 2024, https://www.abim.org/media-center/press-releases/joint-statement-on-dissemination-of-misinformation/.

25. B. Weiss, "Weekend Listening: From McDonalds Drive-Through to Star Harvard Professor: Roland Fryer on Race and Policing, Claudine Gay, and Karma — and Much More," *Free Press,* February 18, 2024, https://www.thefp.com/p/roland-fryer-bari-weiss-honestly-utax-harvard.
26. J. Schuessler et al., "Harvard President Resigns after Mounting Plagiarism Accusations," *New York Times,* January 2, 2024, https://www.nytimes.com/2024/01/02/us/harvard-claudine-gay-resigns.html
27. M. A. Makary and I. Kawachi, "The International Tobacco Strategy," *Journal of the American Medical Association* 280, no. 13 (1998): 1194–95.
28. M. A. Makary et al., "Operating Room Briefings: Working on the Same Page," *Joint Commission Journal on Quality and Patient Safety* 32, no. 6 (June 2006): 351–55.
29. M. A. Makary et al., "Operating Room Briefings and Wrong-Site Surgery," *Journal of the American College of*

Surgeons 204, no. 2 (February 2007): 236–43.
30. E. C. Wick et al., "Implementation of a Surgical Comprehensive Unit-Based Safety Program to Reduce Surgical Site Infections," *Journal of the American College of Surgeons* 215, no. 2 (August 2012): 193–200.
31. M. A. Makary et al., "Frailty as a Predictor of Surgical Outcomes in Older Patients," *Journal of the American College of Surgeons* 210, no. 6 (June 2010): 901–8.
32. G. Kwakye, G. A. Brat, and M. A. Makary, "Green Surgical Practices for Health Care," *Archives of Surgery* 146, no. 2 (February 2011): 131–36.
33. W. E. Bruhn et al., "Prevalence and Characteristics of Virginia Hospitals Suing Patients and Garnishing Wages for Unpaid Medical Bills," *Journal of the American Medical Association* 322, no. 7 (August 2019): 691–92.
34. J. G. R. Paturzo et al., "Trends in Hospital Lawsuits Filed Against Patients for Unpaid Bills Following Published Research About This Activity," *JAMA Network Open* 4, no. 8 (2021) doi:10.1001/jamanetworkopen.2021.21926.

35. S. C. Mathews and M. A. Makary, "Billing Quality Is Medical Quality," *JAMA Network Open* 4, no. 323 (February 2020): 409–10.
36. Z. Damania and P. Teirstein, "Meet the Doc the American Board of Medical Specialties Wants DEAD," *Against Medical Advice* (podcast), February 2, 2018, https://zdoggmd.com/against-medical-advice-035/.

Chapter 12: Imagine

1. V. Prasad et al., "A Decade of Reversal: An Analysis of 146 Contradicted Medical Practices," *Mayo Clinic Proceedings* 88, no. 8 (August 2013): 790–98.
2. A. M. Glenny et al., "Water Fluoridation for the Prevention of Dental Caries," *Cochrane Database of Systematic Reviews,* 6 (June 18, 2015), doi:10.1002/14651858.CD010856.pub2.
3. Centers for Disease Control and Prevention, "Community Water Fluoridation," accessed February 13, 2024, https://www.cdc.gov/fluoridation/index.html.
4. "U.S. States Where Recreational Marijuana Is Legal," Reuters, November 8, 2023, https://www

.reuters.com/world/us/us-states-where-recreational-marijuana-is-legal-2023-05-31/.

5. A. Wnuk, "Is Cannabis Today Really Much More Potent than 50 Years Ago?" *New Scientist,* October 11, 2023, https://www.newscientist.com/article/2396976-is-cannabis-today-really-much-more-potent-than-50-years-ago/.
6. E. Stuyt, "The Problem with the Current High Potency THC Marijuana from the Perspective of an Addiction Psychiatrist," *Missouri Medicine* 115, no. 6 (November–December 2018): 482–86.
7. A. Abouseif, "Adverse Effects of Cannabis Use on Adolescents' Brain," (capstone project, Harvard University, March 17, 2024).
8. G. Gobbi et al., "Association of Cannabis Use in Adolescence and Risk of Depression, Anxiety, and Suicidality in Young Adulthood: A Systematic Review and Meta-Analysis," *JAMA Psychiatry* 76, no. 4 (April 1, 2019): 426–34.
9. N. Castellanos-Ryan et al., "Adolescent Cannabis Use, Change in Neurocognitive Function, and High-School Graduation: A Longitudinal

Study from Early Adolescence to Young Adulthood," *Development and Psychopathology* 29, no. 4 (October 2017): 1253–66.
10. A. M. Jeffers et al., "Association of Cannabis Use with Cardiovascular Outcomes among U.S. Adults," *Journal of the American Heart Association* 13, no. 5 (March 5, 2024), doi:10.1161/JAHA.123.030178.
11. J. Renard et al., "Long-Term Consequences of Adolescent Cannabinoid Exposure in Adult Psychopathology," *Frontiers in Neuroscience* 10, no. 8 (November 2014): 361.
12. L. Degenhardt et al., "Outcomes of Occasional Cannabis Use in Adolescence: 10-Year Follow-Up Study in Victoria, Australia," *British Journal of Psychiatry* 196, no. 4 (April 2010): 290–95.
13. Ibid.
14. Rep. D. LaMalfa, "Cartels Are Turning Our National Forests into a Warzone," The Hill, July 28, 2022, https://thehill.com/opinion/congress-blog/3577673-cartels-are-turning-our-national-forests-into-a-warzone/.
15. B. Warren and M. Clevenger,

"Marijuana Wars: Violent Mexican Drug Cartels Turn Northern California into 'The Wild West,'" *USA Today* and *Louisville Courier Journal,* December 19, 2021.
16. S. Rotella et al., "Gangsters, Money and Murder: How Chinese Organized Crime Is Dominating America's Illegal Marijuana Market," ProPublica, March 14, 2024, https://www.propublica.org/article/chinese-organized-crime-us-marijuana-market.
17. T. F. Doran et al., "Acetaminophen: More Harm than Good for Chickenpox?" *Journal of Pediatrics* 114, no. 6 (June 1989): 1045–8.
18. K. I. Plaisance et al., "Effect of Antipyretic Therapy on the Duration of Illness in Experimental Influenza A, *Shigella sonnei,* and *Rickettsia rickettsii* Infections," *Pharmacotherapy* 20, no. 12 (December 2000): 1417–22.
19. T. A. Mace et al., "Differentiation of CD8+ T Cells into Effector Cells Is Enhanced by Physiological Range Hyperthermia," *Journal of Leukocyte Biology* 90, no. 5 (November 2011): 951–62.
20. C. Lin et al., "Fever Promotes T Lymphocyte Trafficking via a Thermal

Sensory Pathway Involving Heat Shock Protein 90 and α4 Integrins," *Immunity* 50, no. 1 (January 15, 2019): 137–51.e6.
21. Z. Liew et al., "Acetaminophen Use During Pregnancy, Behavioral Problems, and Hyperkinetic Disorders," *JAMA Pediatrics* 168, no. 4 (April 2014): 313–20.
22. J. Cendejas-Hernandez et al., "Paracetamol (Acetaminophen) Use in Infants and Children Was Never Shown to Be Safe for Neurodevelopment: A Systematic Review with Citation Tracking," *European Journal of Pediatrics* 181, no. 5 (May 2022): 1835–57.
23. L. Sensintaffar, "Is Galleri a Miracle Test? It's Too Soon to Say: Early Cancer Detection Isn't the Same as Prevention," *Wall Street Journal,* February 9, 2024.
24. C. Westgate et al., "Early Real-World Experience with a Multi-Cancer Early Detection Test" (paper presented at the American Society of Clinical Oncology Annual Meeting, Chicago, IL, and online, June 2–6, 2023).
25. B. Nicholson et al., "Multi-Cancer Early Detection Test in Symptomatic Patients Referred for Cancer

Investigation in England and Wales (SYMPLIFY): A Large-Scale, Observational Cohort Study," *Lancet* 24, no. 7 (July 2023): 733–43.

26. Sensintaffar, "Is Galleri a Miracle Test?"
27. Westgate et al., "Early Real-World Experience with a Multi-Cancer Early Detection Test."
28. D. Schrag et al., "Blood-Based Tests for Multicancer Early Detection (PATHFINDER): A Prospective Cohort Study," *Lancet* 402, no.10409 (October 2023): 1251–60.
29. J. Smyth, "Quick Blood Tests to Spot Cancer: Will They Help or Harm Patients?" *Financial Times,* May 17, 2023.
30. L. A. Thompson, "European Commission Continues Battle Against Illumina, Orders It to Sell Cancer-Test Developer Grail," Law .com International, October 15, 2023, https://www.law.com /international-edition/2023/10/15 /european-commission-continues -battle-against-illumina-orders -it-to-sell-cancer-test-developer-grail/.
31. Federal Trade Commission, "FTC Orders Illumina to Divest Cancer

Detection Test Maker GRAIL to Protect Competition in Life-Saving Technology Market," press release, April 3, 2023.
32. Icahn Enterprises L.P., "Illumina, Inc.: Case for Change," PowerPoint presentation, Spring 2023, CarlIcahn.com, https://carlicahn.com/wp-content/uploads/2023/04/ILMN-Case-for-Change.pdf.
33. American Cancer Society Cancer Action Network, "Multi-Cancer Early Detection Bill Would Create a Pathway to Coverage for Millions of Cancer Screenings for Medicare Beneficiaries," press release, June 22, 2023.
34. Multicancer Early Detection Consortium, "Closing the Cancer Gap: The Multicancer Early Detection (MCED) Consortium Releases Two New Health Equity Papers," press release, March 2, 2023.
35. J. Tabery, *Tyranny of the Gene: Personalized Medicine and Its Threat to Public Health* (New York: Knopf, 2023).
36. C. Turnbull et al., "GRAIL-Galleri: Why the Special Treatment?" *Lancet* 403, no. 10425 (February 3, 2024): 431–32.

37. J. Park et al., "An Inactivated Multivalent Influenza A Virus Vaccine is Broadly Protective in Mice and Ferrets," *Science Translational Medicine* 14, no. 653 (July 13, 2022), doi:10.1126/scitranslmed.abo2167.
38. U.S. Department of Health and Human Services, National Vaccine Advisory Committee Meeting, Washington, D.C., September 22–23, 2022, https://www.hhs.gov/vaccines/nvac/meetings/2022/09-22/index.html.
39. M. J. Memoli et al., "Evaluation of Antihemagglutinin and Antineuraminidase Antibodies as Correlates of Protection in an Influenza A/H1N1 Virus Healthy Human Challenge Model," *mBio* 7, no. 2 (April 19, 2016), doi:10.1128/mBio.00417-16.
40. B. R. Murphy, J. A. Kasel, and R. M. Chanock, "Association of Serum Anti-Neuraminidase Antibody with Resistance to Influenza in Man," *New England Journal of Medicine* 286 (1972): 1329–32.
41. H. W. Kim et al., "Temperature-Sensitive Mutants of Influenza A Virus: Response of Children to the Influenza A/Hong Kong/68-ts-1[E]

(H3N2) and Influenza A/Udorn/72 -ts-1[E] (H3N2) Candidate Vaccine Viruses and Significance of Immunity to Neuraminidase Antigen," *Pediatric Research* 10, no. 4 (April 1976): 238–42.
42. National Institute of Allergy and Infectious Diseases, "Safety and Immunogenicity of BPL-1357, A BPL-Inactivated, Whole-Virus, Universal Influenza Vaccine," National Institutes of Health Clinical Center, ClinicalTrials.gov, accessed April 4, 2024, https://classic.clinicaltrials.gov/ct2/show/NCT05027932.
43. C. Dun et al., "Sleep Disorders and the Development of Alzheimer's Disease among U.S. Medicare Beneficiaries," *Journal of the American Geriatrics Society* 70, no. 1 (January 2022): 299–301.
44. P. J. Snyder et al., "Effect of Testosterone Treatment on Bone Mineral Density in Men Over 65 Years of Age," *Journal of Clinical Endocrinology and Metabolism* 84, no. 6 (June 1999): 1966–72.
45. P. J. Snyder et al., "Effect of Testosterone Treatment on Body Composition and Muscle Strength in

Men Over 65 Years of Age," *Journal of Clinical Endocrinology and Metabolism* 84, no. 8 (August 1999): 2647–53.

46. X. Cai et al., "Metabolic Effects of Testosterone Replacement Therapy on Hypogonadal Men with Type 2 Diabetes Mellitus: A Systematic Review and Meta-Analysis of Randomized Controlled Trials," *Asian Journal of Andrology* 16, no. 1 (January–February 2014): 146–52.
47. H. Barnes, "Children on Puberty Blockers Saw Mental Health Change: New Analysis," BBC News, September 19, 2023, https://www.bbc.com/news/health-66842352.
48. T. Roush, "UK Bans Puberty Blockers for Minors," Forbes, March 12, 2024, https://www.forbes.com/sites/tylerroush/2024/03/12/uk-bans-puberty-blockers-for-minors/?sh=74b09752a3b3.
49. S. Ruuska et al., "All-Cause and Suicide Mortalities among Adolescents and Young Adults Who Contacted Specialised Gender Identity Services in Finland in 1996–2019: A Register Study," *BMJ Mental Health* 27 (2024), doi:10.1136/bmjment-2023-300940.
50. L. Littman, "Correction: Parent Reports of Adolescents and Young

Adults Perceived to Show Signs of a Rapid Onset of Gender Dysphoria," *PLOS ONE* 14, no. 3 (March 19, 2019), doi:10.1371/journal.pone.0214157.
51. Brown University News, "Updated: Brown Statements on Gender Dysphoria Study," press release, March 19, 2019.
52. M. Grossman, *Lost in Trans Nation* (New York: Skyhorse, 2023).
53. M. Powell, "What Lia Thomas Could Mean for Women's Elite Sports," *New York Times,* May 29, 2022, https://www.nytimes.com/2022/05/29/us/lia-thomas-women-sports.html.
54. J. Kiger, "Prominent Mayo Clinic Physician Sues, Citing Retaliation Over Media Statements, Whistleblowing Report," *Rochester Post-Bulletin,* TwinCities.com, November 17, 2023, https://www.twincities.com/2023/11/17/prominent-mayo-clinic-physician-sues-citing-retaliation-over-media-statements-whistleblowing-report/.
55. Grossman, *Lost in Trans Nation*.
56. Laura Helmuth, X (formerly Twitter), February 16, 2023, 7:26 p.m., https://x.com/laurahelmuth/status/1626377504461127681.
57. V. Murugesh et al., "Puberty Blocker

and Aging Impact on Testicular Cell States and Function" (preprint, posted March 27, 2024), https://www.biorxiv.org/content/10.1101/2024.03.23.586441.
58. J. E. O'Shea et al., "Frenotomy for Tongue-Tie in Newborn Infants," *Cochrane Database of Systematic Reviews* 3 (2017), doi:10.1002/14651858.CD011065.pub2.
59. K. Thomas, S. Kliff, and J. Silver-Greenberg, "Inside the Booming Business of Cutting Babies' Tongues," *New York Times,* December 18, 2023.
60. A. H. Messner et al., "Clinical Consensus Statement: Ankyloglossia in Children," *Otolaryngology–Head and Neck Surgery* 162, no. 5 (2020): 597–611.
61. Information on our Global Appropriateness Measures consortium is available at GAmeasures.com.
62. M. A. Makary et al., "Frailty as a Predictor of Surgical Outcomes in Older Patients," *Journal of the American College of Surgeons* 210, no. 6 (June 2010): 901–8.
63. V. Prasad, "Mammography: Does It Save Lives? The USPSTF Is Incorrect. I Review ALL the Data," YouTube, May 10, 2023, https://www.youtube

.com/watch?v=-9hQO7X1bmU.
64. American Cancer Society, "Limitations of Mammograms," accessed February 18, 2024, https://www.cancer.org/cancer/types/breast-cancer/screening-tests-and-early-detection/mammograms/limitations-of-mammograms.html.
65. G. C. S. Smith and J. P. Pell, "Parachute Use to Prevent Death and Major Trauma Related to Gravitational Challenge: Systematic Review of Randomised Controlled Trials," *BMJ: British Medical Journal* 327 (2003): 1459.
66. W. E. Boden et al., "COURAGE Trial Research Group. Optimal medical therapy with or without PCI for stable coronary disease," *New England Journal of Medicine* 356, no.15 (April 12, 2007): 1503–16.
67. D. L. Sackett, "The Arrogance of Preventive Medicine," *Canadian Medical Association Journal* 167, no. 4 (August 2002): 363–64.
68. D. L. Sackett et al., "Evidence Based Medicine: What It Is and What It Isn't: It's About Integrating Individual Clinical Expertise and the Best External Evidence," *BMJ: British*

Medical Journal 312, no. 7023 (1996): 71–72.
69. R. Habert, "Claude Bernard, the Founder of Modern Medicine," *Cells* 11, no. 10 (May 20, 2022): 1702.

A NOTE ON THE AUTHOR

Dr. Marty Makary is a professor at the Johns Hopkins School of Medicine and a member of the National Academy of Medicine. The author of two *New York Times* bestselling books, *Unaccountable* (Bloomsbury 2012) and *The Price We Pay* (Bloomsbury 2019), he is the recipient of the SABEW Association of Business Journalists's 2020 Best in Business Book Award. A leading voice for physicians in the *Wall Street Journal,* the *New York Times,* and the *Washington Post,* Dr. Makary has been a visiting professor at over 25 medical schools and has published over 300 scientific peer-reviewed articles. A surgeon and public health researcher, he served in leadership at the World Health Organization and currently leads the Evidence-Based Medicine and Public Health Research Group at Johns Hopkins. Dr. Makary is director of the Re-Design of Health Care, a national project to make health care more reliable and affordable, especially for vulnerable populations. His research focuses on the appropriateness of medical care, employer-sponsored health benefits, and the impact of public health efforts. Dr. Makary is the recipient of the Nobility in Science Award from the National Pancreas Foundation and numerous teaching awards. He lives in Baltimore, Maryland.

The employees of Thorndike Press hope you have enjoyed this Large Print book. All our Thorndike Large Print titles are designed for easy reading, and all our books are made to last. Other Thorndike Press Large Print books are available at your library, through selected bookstores, or directly from us.

For information about titles, please visit our website at:

http://gale.cengage.com/thorndike